MW00884618

# Adulting Hard as an Introvert or Highly Sensitive Person

Unleash the Introverted Leader Within, Make Better Small Talk, Set Boundaries, Conquer Anxiety, and Give Yourself Permission to Feel

## Jeffrey C. Chapman

# CONTENTS

# DISCLAIMER

P LEASE KEEP IN MIND that I am not a doctor, mental health professional, or professional therapist. I am an introvert who has spent more than five decades exploring, and learning about the challenges and strengths that introverts and highly sensitive people face. My interest in this subject has led me to collect and share the wisdom and knowledge I've gained over the years.

While I make every effort to provide accurate and useful information, this book should not be used in place of professional medical advice, diagnosis, or treatment. Please consult a qualified healthcare professional if you have any concerns about your mental health or well-being. Remember that everyone's journey is unique, and what works for one person may not work for another.

This book provides general advice and suggestions, but it is critical that you tailor these strategies to your specific needs and circumstances.

# INTRODUCTION

Welcome to Adulting Hard for Introverts and Highly Sensitive People, the definitive guide to navigating adulthood while embracing your unique personality traits. My goal is to provide you with a wealth of information, exercises, and examples in a lighthearted and informative package. I promise never to be condescending, and I'll do my best to make this journey enjoyable and fulfilling.

## Defining Introversion and High Sensitivity

Before we dive into the heart of the matter, let's establish some common ground. From this point forward, I will be using the abbreviations I/HSP to refer to introverts and highly sensitive people.

I/HSP is more than just a label; it represents a rich tapestry of traits and characteristics that shape how people interact with the world around them. It's important to understand these terms as we embark on this journey together.

Introversion is a personality trait that shows up as a preference for quiet, low-stimulation places and a need for alone time to recharge. Introverts often find that being around other people is draining and look for comfort in alone time or small groups. It's important to understand that introversion is a spectrum, and that each person has their own unique mix of introverted traits. Examples of well-known introverts include the brilliant mind of Albert Einstein, the courage of Rosa Parks, and the innovative spirit of Bill Gates.

High sensitivity, on the other hand, means being more aware of emotional, physical, and social stimuli from the outside world. Highly sensitive individuals, or HSPs, possess a remarkable depth of processing and exhibit heightened empathy and sensitivity to their surroundings. It's important to keep in mind that some introverts are also highly sensitive, and vice versa. However, these are two different traits that don't cancel each other out. The term "high sensitivity" was coined by psychologist Dr. Elaine Aron, who estimates that approximately 15-20% of the population possesses this trait.[1]

By understanding these terms and how they are used, we can learn more about how complicated and unique I/HSPs' lives are. In this book, I'll talk about the different aspects, challenges, and strengths of introversion and being highly sensitive. So, let's go on this educational journey together, embracing the uniqueness of I/HSPs and finding the hidden gems in their amazing world.

• • • • • • • • • • •

## What Are the Main Differences Between Introverts and Extroverts?

**Introverts:**

1. Tend to feel energized by spending time alone or in quiet environments.

2. Prefer deep, meaningful conversations with a few close friends.

3. May require more time to process information and make decisions.

4. Often excel in tasks that require focus, reflection, and independent work.

5. Value personal space and boundaries.

6. May feel drained or overwhelmed at large, noisy social gatherings.

---

1. Aron, E. N. (1996). The Highly Sensitive Person: How to Thrive When the World Overwhelms You. Broadway Books.

7. Embrace pastimes and pursuits like reading, writing, and painting that promote solitude or introspection.

8. May be more sensitive to external stimuli, such as loud noises or bright lights.

**Extroverts**:

1. Tend to feel energized by spending time with others and engaging in social activities.

2. Enjoy meeting new people and engaging in small talk or group conversations.

3. May process information and make decisions more quickly.

4. Often excel in tasks that require teamwork, collaboration, and communication.

5. Value social connections and shared experiences.

6. Thrive in large, lively social gatherings and events.

7. Enjoy hobbies and activities that involve socializing or group participation, such as team sports or clubs.

8. May be more comfortable in stimulating environments and adapt more easily to noise and activity.

Remember that introversion and extroversion are two ends of a spectrum; many people display characteristics of both introverts and extroverts. This is just a short list meant to give you a sense of the broad categories of personality.

· · · · ● · ● · · ·

## The Unique Challenges and Strengths of Introverts and Highly Sensitive People in Adulting

Adulting is difficult for everyone, but introverts and highly sensitive people face unique challenges and strengths. Let's explore a few examples:

## Challenges

- **Socializing and Networking:** I/HSPs may find socializing and networking events exhausting or even anxiety-inducing.

- **Workplace Stress:** Open office environments, constant collaboration, and high-pressure situations can be particularly taxing for I/HSPs.

- **Misunderstandings:** People may misinterpret introversion or high sensitivity as shyness, aloofness, or even rudeness.

## Strengths

- **Deep Thinking:** I/HSPs are often reflective and capable of deep thought, making them excellent problem solvers and critical thinkers.

- **Empathy:** Both I/HSPs tend to be empathetic and understanding, which can be valuable in relationships and the workplace.

- **Creativity:** I/HSPs frequently have a rich inner world, which can lead to unique creative pursuits and hobbies.

In this book, I'll address these challenges and strengths head on, offering practical advice, exercises, and examples to help you thrive as an adult. Whether you identify as an introvert or highly sensitive, I'll discuss:

- How to thrive in social situations,

- How to handle money responsibly,

- How to take care of yourself,

- How to develop as a person,

- What it's like to build a safe space at home,

- How to travel and see the world,

- How to adapt to new situations, and much more.

Let's take this exciting journey together and learn what it takes to be an introvert and an HSP in the real world.

# CHAPTER ONE

# EMBRACING YOUR INNER INTROVERT AND HIGHLY SENSITIVE SELF

## Unraveling the Myths Around Introversion and High Sensitivity

T HERE ARE MANY MYTHS and misconceptions about I/HSPs that can make it difficult for us to embrace our unique characteristics. Let's bust some of the most common myths to help you understand yourself and others better:

1. **Myth: Introverts are antisocial hermits.**

   The truth is that introverts prefer quality over quantity when it comes to social interactions. While we might not be the life of the party, we are more likely to have a deep, meaningful conversation with you in a quiet corner of the room. For example, I enjoy having deep conversations with my close friends over dinner. I would rather be in this intimate setting than at a loud and crowded party.

2. **Myth: Highly sensitive people are just overly emotional crybabies.**

   In reality, HSPs have a heightened ability to perceive and process emotions, which can make them more empathetic and understanding. They're not just upset about the spilled milk; they're feeling the milk's pain as it splatters on the floor. For example, Tom, an HSP, may be moved to tears by a powerful movie scene, but his empathetic nature also allows him to provide emotional support to his friends in times of need.

3. **Myth: Introverts don't like people.**

   Introverts enjoy socializing, but we also need time alone to recharge. Imagine us as battery-operated social butterflies; we can fly from one gathering to the next, making new friends and acquaintances, but we'll need to recharge in our cocoon every so often.

4. **Myth: Highly sensitive people are weak and fragile.**

   On the contrary! Because of their ability to deeply process experiences and emotions, HSPs are frequently very resilient. They may need a little more time to recover from life's curveballs, but once they do, they are stronger than ever. As an example, Michael, an HSP, is dealing with a difficult personal challenge. He needs time to work through his feelings and experiences, but he eventually comes out on the other side of the ordeal more confident and capable than before.

· • • ● • ● • • ·

# Self-Discovery

## Identifying Your Strengths and Weaknesses

Now that we've dispelled some common myths about I/HSPs, it's time to do some introspection. Understanding your own strengths and weaknesses can help you navigate adulthood with greater self-awareness and confidence. Here are some pointers to get you started:

1. **Assess your energy levels.** Do you find yourself exhausted or revitalized after spending time with others? How do you feel when you're alone—refreshed and ready to go, or lonely and isolated? You can learn more about your introverted or extroverted tendencies by analyzing your energy preferences. For example, I usually feel drained after attending large networking events. However, I feel successful and energized when I have one-on-one meetings or small group discussions with colleagues.

2. **Reflect on past experiences.** Think about the times you felt the most at ease and successful. What did they all have in common? On the other hand, think about times when you had trouble. Patterns can help you figure out what your strengths and weaknesses are.

3. **Take a personality test.** Although not 100% accurate, tools such as the Myers-Briggs (MBTI) or the Highly Sensitive Person Scale may offer insight into your personality traits and help you better understand yourself. Taking a personality test can be a fun and interesting way to find out more about who you are and what makes you unique. Even though no personality test is perfect or covers everything, the Myers-Briggs Type Indicator (MBTI) and the Highly Sensitive Person Scale can tell you a lot about your habits and preferences.

**Myers-Briggs Type Indicator (MBTI)**

The MBTI is a popular tool for figuring out a person's personality. It sorts people into one of 16 types based on their preferences in four areas:

1. **Extroversion (E) vs. Introversion (I):** This scale shows how you gain and lose energy, such as whether you get more energy from being around other people or from being alone.

2. **Sensing (S) vs. Intuition (N):** This scale looks at how you collect and look at data. It looks at how much you focus on concrete facts and details or how much you use abstract ideas and patterns.

3. **Thinking (T) vs. Feeling (F):** This scale evaluates your decision-making process—whether you prioritize logic and objectivity or emotions and personal values.

4. **Judging (J) vs. Perceiving (P):** This scale measures how you approach structure and organization—whether you prefer to plan and make decisions or remain open and adaptable to new information.

Learning your MBTI personality type can help you better understand yourself, others, your communication preferences, and your career options.

**Highly Sensitive Person Scale**

The Highly Sensitive Person (HSP) Scale is a self-assessment tool that measures sensory-processing sensitivity, which affects 15-20% of the population. Highly sensitive people are more affected by sensory stimuli, process information more deeply, and have stronger emotional reactions.

Taking the HSP Scale can help you identify if you are a highly sensitive person and give you insight into what it's like to be one. If you know how sensitive you are, you can modify your surroundings and habits to suit your preferences.

**Other Personality Tests**

There are many other personality tests and assessments, like the **Big Five Personality Test**, the **Enneagram**, and the **DISC assessment**. Each test gives you a different view of your personality traits, preferences, and habits, which can help you learn more about yourself and how you interact with others.

Remember that personality tests can be helpful, but they can't tell you everything. People are complicated and have many sides, so no one test can tell you everything about yourself. You should use these assessments as guides for self-improvement, but you should never reduce yourself to a single score.

· · · · ●·●· · ·

## Celebrating Your Unique Personality

Celebrate who you are in all your singular glory, whether you identify as an introvert or a highly sensitive person. Here's how:

1. **Value your strengths.** Introverts are usually good at listening, being empathetic, and thinking deeply, while HSPs are very intuitive, empathetic, and creative. Recognize and value these qualities, and let them shine in your everyday life. *Emily is a highly sensitive person. As a graphic designer, she uses her intuition and creativity to do well in her job.*

2. **Accept your quirks.** Maybe you're the type who needs to use earplugs in the

theater or who prefers to spend Friday nights curled up with a book instead of going out. That's totally acceptable! Recognize that it is precisely your peculiarities that define you. *To recharge during his lunch breaks, Kevin, an introvert, knows exactly where to find the most peaceful corners of a busy café.*

3. **Don't compare yourself to others.** Keep in mind that this is not a competition; everyone has their own set of skills and abilities. Focus on your own journey and be proud of how much you've grown and what you've done.

• • • ●•• ● • •• •

## Acknowledging Your Unique Experiences

Life as an introvert or HSP is filled with its own set of experiences. Acknowledge these experiences and learn from them:

1. **Embrace the awkward moments.** Let's be honest: we've all been in awkward situations. You may be more susceptible to them as an introvert or HSP, and that's fine! Rather than ruminating on your awkwardness, try to laugh it off and keep in mind that it happens to the best of us. *Sarah, an introvert, spills her drink on a stranger after she bumps into them at a party. She laughs it off and starts a conversation with the stranger, turning the awkward situation into a chance to meet a new friend.*

2. **Learn from your challenges.** Individuals who are highly sensitive or introverted may have difficulty navigating everyday life. Take advantage of this difficulty to learn something new about yourself and acquire traits like assertiveness, boundary-setting, or self-care. *For instance, Lily has a hard time focusing at work because of all the background noise. To overcome this obstacle, she has started wearing noise-cancelling headphones and taking frequent breaks in a quiet area.*

3. **Celebrate your victories.** Whether it's making a new friend, making it through a networking event, or just finding a quiet place where you can relax, it's important to recognize and celebrate your accomplishments, no matter how

small they may seem. *Even though he was nervous, Alex, an introvert, gave a great presentation at the conference. He gives himself a night in to reflect on his success and enjoy some downtime.*

The first step toward accepting your introverted or highly sensitive self is to learn the truth about these personality traits, identify your own strengths and weaknesses, and accept the value of your own life experiences. Always remember that the things that make you special can also be your greatest strengths as you face the challenges and reap the rewards of adulthood.

# CHAPTER TWO

## NAVIGATING SOCIAL LIFE AND RELATIONSHIPS

### Friends and Family

EVERY DAY IS AN epic struggle for an introvert like me to get by in a world that seems to favor extroverts. You see, I enjoy spending time with my loved ones, but man, do I ever tire from attending social gatherings.

I'll set the scene: it's Friday night, and I have plans to attend a friend's birthday party. Since I care deeply about this friend, I am looking forward to it; however, I can't help but dread the packed house. And not just any folks, but the chatty sort who seem to flit from one conversation to the next like sociable flies on a caffeine high.

So, I get dressed in my go-to outfit, which is casual but still puts me in a good mood, and I chant to myself, "You can do this!" as I walk out the door.

The party's overwhelming atmosphere of noise, bright lights, and countless people all hit me like a wave the moment I stepped inside. It's as if I'm a fish out of water, struggling for air and looking desperately for a way to get out. But no, I remind myself, "You can do this!"

When I see a friendly face, I immediately strike up a conversation using my tried and true arsenal of conversation starters. "How are things at the office?", "Have you read any good books recently?", "Any good movies lately?"

I'm really getting into it, but then it happens: I hit a mental block and can't think of anything else to say. Cue the awkward silence.

But I refuse to be defeated. I nod, smile, and head for the safety of the snack table. While stuffing my face full of chips and dip, I survey the room like a general sizing up his troops. When I see another familiar face, I know it's time for round two.

I weave in and out of conversations and seek refuge in the restroom for brief periods of quiet throughout the evening. At one point, I'm cornered by a bubbly extroverted person who wants to hear about my day, my loved ones, and my plans to rule the world (okay, maybe not the last one).

The longer the night goes on, the more I feel my strength ebbing away. It's as if a neon sign reading "Low Battery" were attached to my social battery, signaling that it's time to leave. I say my goodbyes, thank my host, and sneak out into the dark, enjoying the peace and quiet.

As I drive home, I can't help but chuckle at the absurdity of my introverted existence. Although I sometimes find it difficult to interact with others, I wouldn't change my introverted personality. It's a big part of what makes me unique, and I've learned to be proud of it even when it seems like the world around me wasn't built with me in mind.

· · · ● · ● · · ·

## Building a Support Network

I/HSPs often struggle to find a balance between their need for solitude and their desire to form meaningful relationships with others. As an introvert or highly sensitive person, you may feel like Schrödinger's cat, desiring both solitude and company. But don't worry! It's entirely possible to build a support network that accommodates your unique needs.

- **Quality over quantity:** Focus on developing a small but strong circle of friends and family who truly understand and appreciate your personality.

- **Establish a mutual understanding:** Communicate openly with your loved ones about your introversion or high sensitivity. This will help them understand your need for alone time and set the stage for a more supportive relationship.

- **Stay connected:** Make regular, low-key plans to maintain your relationships, such as going for a walk, having a quiet dinner, or attending a small gathering. This way, you can foster meaningful connections without overstimulating your senses.

Let's say you've been invited to a party at a friend's place. You can't wait to see some old friends, but you're also planning to sneak out early so you can have some quiet time to yourself at home. As an I/HSP, you value these meaningful connections, but you also recognize the importance of recharging your batteries.

After getting there, you have a great time chatting it up with your pals and taking in the atmosphere. However, as the night progresses and the volume increases, you begin to feel exhausted. It's at this point that you decide to put your exit plan into action.

You politely inform your friends that you're getting tired and need to go home to rest. Being understanding and supportive, they appreciate your honesty and wish you a good night. You leave the gathering with a sense of fulfillment, knowing you've nurtured your friendships without compromising your need for self-care and rejuvenation.

· · · · ●·●· · ·

## Creating Meaningful Connections

For an I/HSP, making and maintaining meaningful connections is essential. If you want to make and keep these connections, consider the following methods:

- **Listen with intent:** I/HSPs are often great listeners, which can be a powerful tool for fostering connection. As the saying goes, "we have two ears and one mouth, so we can listen twice as much as we speak." You can make people feel valued and heard if you listen to them carefully and talk to them with empathy.

- **Be authentic:** Embrace your true self and resist the urge to conform to societal expectations. By being authentic, you'll draw people with the same values as your unique qualities.

- **Go deep:** Engage in deeper conversations that go beyond small talk. Ask open-ended questions that encourage others to share their experiences, thoughts, and emotions.

· · · · ●· ● · · ·

## Communicating Effectively

In general, but especially for I/HSPs, good communication skills are crucial to the success of any relationship.

For I/HSPs, interacting with others can bring up a wide range of feelings and worries. On one hand, they may appreciate the opportunity to connect deeply and engage in meaningful conversations. They have a knack for connecting with others through active listening and sympathetic understanding. On the other hand, they may fear being misunderstood or judged for their unique traits and preferences. They may be anxious about expressing themselves clearly, especially in challenging or stimulating situations. Since I/HSPs typically need more time to process information and formulate responses, they may also feel overwhelmed by the demands of social interactions. Despite these obstacles, they are typically drawn to open and honest forms of communication where they can be themselves and build meaningful relationships.

**Here are some ways to improve your communication skills:**

- **Choose your medium:** If face-to-face conversations are too overwhelming, consider alternative forms of communication, such as texting, emailing, or video calls. This can help reduce anxiety and allow for more thoughtful responses.

- **Practice assertiveness:** As an I/HSP, it's essential to express your needs and set boundaries. Learn to say "no" when necessary and communicate your preferences clearly and respectfully.

- **Develop nonverbal communication skills:** Body language, facial expressions, and gestures can convey messages just as powerfully as words. Pay attention to your nonverbal cues and the cues of others to enhance your communication skills.

· · · ● · ● · ● · · ·

## Setting Boundaries

Setting boundaries is especially important for I/HSPs because it allows them to maintain their mental and emotional well-being in a world that frequently values extroversion and constant social interaction. Setting clear boundaries enables them to communicate their needs, preferences, and limits to others, allowing them to participate in social situations without feeling overwhelmed or drained. They can also create a healthy balance between social activities and personal time by setting boundaries, which is essential for recharging their energy and maintaining a sense of inner peace. Additionally, establishing limits enables I/HSPs to cultivate more genuine relationships, as they are free to be themselves without worrying about how others will react. As a result, they are able to feel more secure and happy in their relationships thanks to the protective effect of boundaries.

Picture a workplace where a number of employees have established a lunchtime ritual of meeting in the break room. There is a buzz of activity as they chat, tell tales, and make jokes with one another. For an extrovert, this lively social setting may be enjoyable and even reinvigorating, providing a much-needed break from work and an opportunity to connect with others.

This same environment, however, may feel overwhelming and overstimulating to an introvert or HSP, making it difficult for them to relax and recharge during their lunch break. They might prefer a quieter, more serene setting where they can enjoy their meal and reflect in peace. In this situation, an introvert or HSP might politely excuse themselves from the group, explain that they need some quiet time to recharge, and find a peaceful spot to spend their lunch break. By setting this limit, they can honor their need for solitude and take care of their health, even if they work in a place that is more suited to people who like to be around other people.

**Here are some guidelines for establishing limits with loved ones:**

- **Be proactive:** Communicate your boundaries early in a relationship to avoid misunderstandings and resentment later on.

- **Be specific:** Clearly state your needs, such as the amount of alone time you require or your preference for quiet environments.

- **Reinforce your boundaries:** If your boundaries are crossed, calmly reassert them and remind the person of your preferences.

· · · · • · • · · ·

## Romantic Relationships

### Attracting the Right Partner

When dating, it's important to be comfortable with your own introverted or highly sensitive nature.

I/HSPs may face some unique challenges in romantic relationships that others may not. For example, they are more susceptible to sensory overload and can become overwhelmed in environments with loud noises, bright lights, or strong smells. As a result, date ideas like concerts or crowded bars may become less appealing or even uncomfortable for them.

Another aspect is their desire for deep, meaningful connections in their romantic relationships, which may be harder to find. They may have difficulty with small talk and prefer to jump right into conversations that have more depth and emotional intimacy. Because of this, it may be difficult to strike up a conversation with people who are more comfortable with light, casual topics.

I/HSPs also need more personal space and solitude to recharge their batteries, which can be difficult to achieve in a relationship. They may have to navigate their partner's expectations and social needs while also making time for themselves. If their partner is not fully aware of their needs, this balancing act can sometimes lead to misunderstandings or conflicts.

It's also possible for I/HSPs to be overly sensitive to their partners' emotions and reactions, leading them to take things personally or worry unnecessarily. In addition to promoting empathy and understanding, heightened sensitivity may also add stress and anxiety to a relationship.

Navigating these unique challenges requires open communication, understanding, and mutual respect between partners, as well as a willingness to embrace each other's differences and grow together.

**The following is a list of some advice that can help you attract the ideal partner for you:**

1. **Be yourself, but better:** I know, it's cliché. But really, who else are you going to be? Embrace your introversion or high sensitivity like a superhero wearing a cape (even if it's an invisible one). Flaunt your unique qualities like you're strutting down the catwalk of life.

2. **Choose the right environment, not the "rite" one:** Forget the rituals of crowded bars and noisy clubs. Instead, find groups that share your interests and values, such as a book club where you can talk about the latest page-turner, an art class where you can express yourself through creation, or a hiking club where you can enjoy the peace and quiet of nature. These settings tend to attract those with similar interests and values, and fewer wild party animals.

3. **Slow and steady wins the race (and the heart):** You're an introvert or HSP, not a cheetah, so don't act like one! You should go at your own pace because it takes time to establish rapport and trust. Let your relationships mature naturally; after all, like a good bottle of wine or cheese, they only get better with age.

4. **Embrace your inner comedian:** Humor can be a fantastic icebreaker, even for

I/HSPs. So go ahead, crack a joke or share a funny story. Laughter is not only the best medicine; it's also a fantastic way to bond with potential partners.

5. **Be a conversation ninja:** Make the most of your introvert or HSP superpowers by asking open-ended questions and actively listening to your conversation partner. You will not only come across as a great conversationalist, but you will also form deeper bonds with those you meet.

Remember that your introversion or heightened sensitivity is a strength, not a flaw. Accept your unique characteristics, and you'll find someone who appreciates you for the amazing person you are.

• • • • •• • •• • •

## Balancing Your Needs with Your Partner's

When dating another introvert or HSP, the dynamics can be quite complementary because both partners are likely to understand each other's need for solitude and quiet time. In such relationships, both individuals may enjoy spending quality time together in low-key settings or participating in activities that do not necessitate large social gatherings. They can connect over their shared love of depth and emotional connection and their appreciation for calm and peaceful surroundings.

However, dating another introvert or HSP can present difficulties, such as the risk of both partners becoming overly withdrawn or isolated. Both people need to find a balance between their introverted tendencies and their need for social interaction and outside stimulation.

When an I/HSP dates an extrovert, on the other hand, things can be both exciting and hard. The outgoing partner can bring energy and a sense of adventure to the relationship, which can encourage the introvert or HSP to leave their comfort zone and try new things. This can be advantageous for personal development and broadening one's horizons.

But when an I/HSP has a partner who is more outgoing, their different needs can sometimes cause misunderstandings or fights. For example, the introverted partner may feel drained by constant social activities, while the outgoing partner may feel unfulfilled or restless without regular social stimulation. In these situations, it's important for both partners to talk openly about their wants and needs and find ways to find a balance that works for both of them.

In both cases, the key to a good relationship is to understand and respect each other's needs, talk to each other honestly, and be willing to change and grow together.

A good romantic relationship is built on understanding and compromise. Here's how to make sure both of your needs are met:

- **Communicate openly:** Talk to your partner about how you feel, what you need, and what your limits are. Open communication will help you both understand each other's unique personalities and create a supportive environment.

- **Find common ground:** Find common hobbies and interests that you and your partner enjoy, so you can spend quality time together without compromising your needs.

- **Respect each other's differences.** You should accept and value your partner's unique qualities and needs, and they should do the same for you. Remember that your differences can bring out the best in each other and make your relationship stronger.

• • • ● • ● • • •

## Maintaining a Healthy and Fulfilling Relationship

The following are some suggestions for maintaining a happy and healthy romantic partnership:

- **Prioritize self-care:** Take care of yourself through regular activities such as exercise, meditation, or hobbies. This will help you stay grounded and better equipped to handle the challenges of a relationship.

- **Support each other's growth:** Make sure your partner is growing and developing as well, and seek their support in your own development as well. In order for a relationship to be healthy, both parties must be committed to growing together.

- **Create shared rituals:** Create habits and customs that strengthen your relationship, such as a weekly date night, daily walks, or cooking dinner together.

· · · · ● · ● · · ·

## Conflict Resolution and Communication

Disagreements are unavoidable in any relationship, but they can be especially difficult for I/HSPs.

I/HSPs may find conflict especially difficult because they process emotions more deeply and may be more sensitive to criticism or negative feedback. As a result, conflicts can feel overwhelming or emotionally draining for them, making it difficult to engage in productive discussions and find resolutions.

An introvert or HSP, for example, may become irritated if their partner criticizes them for not being more outgoing or sociable. This criticism can be deeply personal because it touches on an inherent aspect of their personality. In response, they might pull away or shut down so they don't have to deal with the emotional turmoil any longer.

Similarly, people who are very sensitive can be more aware of their partner's feelings and nonverbal cues when they are fighting. They might notice small changes in the way their partner talks or moves, which could make them feel worse. For example, if their partner shows signs of frustration or anger, an HSP might take on those feelings and feel even worse, making it hard to keep talking calmly and logically.

To deal with these problems, I/HSPs need to learn how to communicate well and how to settle conflicts. They can train themselves to listen actively, empathize, and speak up for themselves without becoming overly emotional. It's also important for them to be in tune with their own needs and realize when they need a break from the conversation to gather their thoughts and feelings.

On the other hand, their partner should understand their unique needs and try to talk to them in a supportive and respectful way, keeping in mind that an introvert or HSP might need a different way to solve a problem than someone else. Partners can strengthen their relationship and better weather the storms of conflict by working together and maintaining open lines of communication.

**A few suggestions for mending fences and keeping the lines of communication open:**

- **Stay calm:** If you have a fight with someone, take a deep breath and try to stay calm. This will help keep things from getting worse and give you a chance to think more clearly.

- **Use "I" statements:** Tell your partner how you feel and what you need without blaming or accusing them. For example, instead of saying "You always make me go to parties," say "I feel overwhelmed when we have too many social plans."

- **Seek understanding:** Listen to your partner and try to see things from their point of view. By being aware of each other's feelings and needs, you can work together to find a solution that makes everyone happy.

• • • ● • ● • • •

## Socializing and Networking

### Tips for Attending Social Events

As mentioned above, I/HSPs can feel anxious at social events for a number of different reasons. The crowds, the pressure to make small talk, and the need to talk to a lot of people can make them feel overwhelmed and tired. Also, I/HSPs may worry that people will judge them for being quiet or shy, which can make their anxiety worse.

Having a few conversation starters in mind can help ease some of the stress and make social events easier to handle. These can help break the ice so you can start talking to people and making connections without feeling too overwhelmed.

**Here are some ideas for conversation starters:**

1. "I love your outfit! Where did you get it?"

2. "How do you know the host/hostess?"

3. "Have you been on any exciting trips lately?"

4. "What's your favorite thing to do in your free time?"

5. "Did you catch the latest episode of [popular TV show]? What did you think?"

6. "I've been looking for a new book to read. Do you have any recommendations?"

7. "What's your favorite local restaurant or cafe?"

8. "Have you seen any good movies recently?"

9. "Do you have any plans for the upcoming weekend or holiday?"

10. "I've been trying to find new hobbies to explore. What do you enjoy doing?"

When you go to parties or other social gatherings with a few conversation starters in mind, you'll feel more at ease and confident in your ability to strike up conversations and make new friends. If you feel yourself becoming overwhelmed, remind yourself that it is acceptable to take breaks and step away for a moment to recharge. Prepare yourself and take care of yourself before going to any social event, and you'll have a much better chance of having a positive experience.

· • • ● • ● • • • ·

## Overcoming Social Anxiety

Social anxiety is a fear of being around other people and a constant fear of being judged, embarrassed, or humiliated in front of them. The symptoms can range from mild to severe and affect each person differently.

Mild symptoms may include a slight feeling of nervousness or unease in social situations, avoiding eye contact sometimes, or being hesitant to start conversations. In these situations, the person might still be able to get along with other people, but it might be awkward.

As social anxiety gets worse, people may sweat a lot, have a fast heartbeat, tremble, have trouble speaking, or even have panic attacks. In these cases, the person's fear of social situations can be so strong that they may try to avoid social events or anything else that might make them anxious.

Social anxiety can be crippling for people who have it because it can make it hard for them to make friends, do everyday things, and reach their personal and professional goals. In the worst cases, social anxiety can cause people to avoid other people, become depressed, and have a much lower quality of life overall.

According to the Anxiety and Depression Association of America (ADAA), social anxiety disorder affects approximately 15 million adults in the United States, or 6.8% of the population[1].

Social anxiety is common and hard to deal with, but people can learn to control their symptoms and have a more fulfilling social life with the right support, coping skills, and, if needed, professional help.

For I/HSPs, social anxiety can be a significant obstacle. Here are some strategies to help you overcome social anxiety:

- **Challenge negative thoughts:** Identify and reframe negative thoughts that

---

1. Anxiety and Depression Association of America. (n.d.). Social anxiety Disorder. https://adaa.org/understanding-anxiety/social-anxiety-disorder

contribute to social anxiety, such as "I'll embarrass myself" or "People will judge me." Replace these thoughts with more realistic and positive ones.

- **Practice relaxation techniques:** Use relaxation methods like deep breathing, progressive muscle relaxation, or mindfulness meditation, to help calm your nerves before and during social situations.

- **Start small:** You can get used to being around people by going to smaller gatherings or doing things that interest you. Gradually expose yourself to more challenging situations as you build confidence and resilience.

- **Seek professional help:** If your social anxiety has a big impact on your life, you might want to talk to a therapist or counselor to help you find ways to deal with it and figure out what's causing it.

· • • ●•● • • ·

## Making Genuine Connections Without Overextending Yourself

As an I/HSP, it's important to make real connections while also taking care of yourself and respecting your need for solitude. Here are some tips for striking the right balance:

- **Prioritize meaningful interactions:** Focus on making deep, meaningful connections with a small group of people instead of trying to make friends with a lot of people.

- **Schedule downtime:** Set aside time after social events to relax and recharge. This will help you keep up your energy and keep you from getting burned out.

- **Set boundaries:** Be clear about what you want and what you need when you talk to other people. Tell them when you need time to yourself or want to hang out in a quieter, more private place.

- **Learn to say "no":** When you need time to yourself, practice politely declining invitations or requests. Remember that it's important to put yourself and your mental health first.

With these tips and strategies, introverts and people with high sensitivity can handle social life and relationships without changing who they are. Accept your strengths, talk openly, and put yourself first if you want to make meaningful connections and have a well-rounded social life.

# CHAPTER THREE

## ADULTING HARD IN THE WORKPLACE

## Choosing the Right Career – Identifying your passions and interests

T HE FIRST STEP IN choosing the right career is to figure out what you're interested in and what you're passionate about. Take some time to reflect on what activities and topics genuinely excite you. Think about what you like to do in your free time and what you're naturally drawn to. Remember that your interests and passions may change over time, and that's fine. Your career should be able to evolve with you.

Work environments that encourage introspection and individual achievement are ideal for introverts. This could be the case in the arts, in academia, or in any field where critical thinking is highly valued.

It's important to ask yourself some deep questions as you begin the process of figuring out what you're truly interested in. Using these questions, you can learn more about what drives and fascinates you. Spend some time thinking about each inquiry and writing down your responses. Don't worry about getting it wrong; this activity is meant to help you learn more about yourself and your own particular set of strengths and weaknesses.

**Tips for Figuring Out What You're Really Interested In:**

1. **What activities or tasks make time fly by?** Think about times when you get

so involved in what you're doing that you forget how much time has passed. Most of the time, these things show a strong interest or passion.

2. **What topics or subjects do you enjoy learning about?** Think about the things you're naturally interested in and like to learn more about or talk about with others.

3. **When you were a child, what did you dream of becoming?** Think about what you wanted to be when you were young and how that might relate to what you want to do now.

4. **What do you enjoy doing in your free time?** Hobbies and other things you do for fun can tell you a lot about what you like and what you care about.

5. **What are the common themes in the books, movies, or articles you enjoy?** By looking at the themes and topics that keep drawing your attention, you can find areas of interest.

6. **What issues or causes are you passionate about?** Think about the problems or injustices that motivate you to take action or get involved.

7. **What skills or talents do you possess that bring you joy?** Think about what makes you special and how your skills and interests might go together.

8. **If money and time were not a concern, what would you spend your days doing?** This question can help you figure out what activities and pursuits really make you happy and excited, without any practical constraints.

9. **Who are your role models, and what about them inspires you?** Consider the qualities, accomplishments, or passions of the people you admire and how they might relate to your own interests.

10. **What are your core values?** Understanding your values can help you identify the passions and interests that align with your beliefs and priorities.

Keep an eye out for themes and trends as you think about these questions. These realizations can help you select a profession that is a good fit for your interests and values, leading to greater happiness and success in your working life.

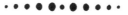

# Assessing job environments that suit your personality

If you are an I/HSP, you should think about the work environment when choosing a job. You should look for places that give you a good mix of social interaction and solitude so that you can recharge when you need to. Think about things like how loud it is, how much teamwork is needed, and the overall culture of the organization.

**What are the best jobs for introverts and HSP's?**

While there isn't a definitive list of "best jobs" for I/HSPs, certain jobs tend to align well with their needs and strengths. Everyone is different, so the ideal job for one I/HSP might not be the same for another. HSPs and introverts often thrive in these careers:

1. **Writer/Editor:** Writing and editing provide opportunities for deep focus, solitude, and creative expression, all of which are attractive qualities for I/HSPs.

2. **Graphic Designer:** Working as a graphic designer allows I/HSPs to use their creativity and attention to detail in a relatively independent setting.

3. **Researcher:** Whether in academia, a private company, or a government institution, research roles often involve deep focus and analysis, which can be appealing to I/HSPs.

4. **Counselor/Therapist:** I/HSPs are known for their empathetic listening skills and ability to understand others' emotions, making them well-suited for roles in counseling and therapy.

5. **Accountant:** I/HSPs who enjoy working with numbers and have strong analytical skills may find satisfaction in a career as an accountant.

6. **Librarian/Archivist:** These roles involve organizing and managing information, often in a quiet, structured environment, which can be appealing to I/HSPs.

7. **IT Specialist:** Careers in information technology, such as software development or network administration, often involve problem-solving and working independently, making them suitable for I/HSPs.

8. **Animal Caretaker:** Working with animals, such as in a veterinary clinic or animal shelter, can provide a nurturing environment where I/HSPs can use their empathy and sensitivity to care for creatures that often communicate non-verbally.

9. **Scientist:** Whether in the field of biology, chemistry, physics, or another scientific discipline, I/HSPs can thrive in roles that involve deep analysis and problem-solving.

10. **Medical Laboratory Technologist:** This career involves analyzing medical samples and conducting tests in a lab setting, often with limited direct patient interaction, which can be ideal for I/HSPs who are interested in healthcare.

It's important to keep in mind that the "best" job for an introvert or HSP will depend on their interests, strengths, and preferences. When looking for a job, think about what you're passionate about and what kind of work environment would be best for you as an introvert or HSP.

**And, what are the worst jobs for introverts and HSP's?**

It is important to remember that the word "worst" is subjective and means something different to each person. However, I/HSPs may find certain professions especially taxing due to their personality types. These jobs can be stressful for I/HSPs because of the high volume of social interaction, the high intensity of sensory stimulation, or the high pressure of the situation. Some examples of careers that may not be a good fit are:

1. **Sales Representative:** Sales positions usually call for constant socialization, persuasion, and extroverted behavior, which can be draining for I/HSPs.

2. **Public Relations Specialist:** Managing an organization's public image is part of public relations. This often requires frequent networking and communication with the public and media, which can be overwhelming for introverts and people with high sensitivity.

3. **Event Planner:** Event planning is a stressful job that requires a lot of multitasking, social interaction, and coordination, which can be difficult for I/HSPs who prefer a more structured, low-key environment.

4. **Customer Service Representative:** Customer service positions require constant interaction with customers, which can be mentally and emotionally draining for I/HSPs.

5. **Telemarketer:** Like sales, telemarketing involves calling potential customers without their permission. This can be hard for I/HSPs who may have trouble being assertive and dealing with rejection.

6. **Flight Attendant:** Flight attendants have to talk to people in a small, noisy space and handle stressful situations, which can be hard for introverts and people with high sensitivity.

7. **Bartender:** Working as a bartender means working in a loud, chaotic place with a lot of people, which can be overwhelming for introverts and people with high sensitivity.

8. **Restaurant Server:** Servers have to talk to customers, do more than one thing at once, and deal with a fast-paced, noisy environment. This can be hard for introverts and people with high sensitivity.

9. **Emergency Medical Technician (EMT):** EMTs work under a lot of stress and have to make quick decisions while giving medical care. This can be hard for I/HSPs, who can feel overwhelmed in these situations.

10. **Broadcast Journalist:** This job involves reporting live news, which can be stressful and requires a strong on-camera presence. Introverts and people with high sensitivity may not be good fits for this job.

It's important to remember that these are generalizations and that I/HSPs can be successful and happy in any job, depending on their strengths and interests. The key is to figure out what your needs and preferences are and then choose a career that fits them best.

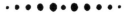

# Job hunting and interviews

People who are shy or highly sensitive may feel like job hunting and interviews are like walking through a minefield of social expectations and situations that make them feel anxious. We have to get out of our comfort zones a lot during the process, whether we're networking to find job openings, listing our accomplishments on a resume, or selling ourselves to potential employers in an interview. I/HSPs may find it hard to stand up for themselves, talk confidently about their achievements, or make a lasting impression in high-pressure situations. But with practice, self-awareness, and a focus on our unique strengths, we can learn to approach job hunting and interviews with more confidence and resilience. This will help us get opportunities that match our skills and passions.

Here are some tips to help you stand out and improve your chances of landing that dream job:

- **Research the company:** Do your homework on the business to learn about its culture and values before you apply for a job or go to an interview. This will help you determine if it's a good fit for your personality and needs.

- **Highlight your strengths:** If you're an introvert or highly sensitive person, you probably excel at things like active listening, empathy, and concentration. Emphasize these strengths in your resume, cover letter, and interviews.

- **Practice:** Be ready for interviews by practicing answers to typical questions. As a result, you'll have a better sense of self-worth and be able to express yourself more clearly.

- **Ask questions:** Inquire about the work environment and company culture during interviews. This will help you determine whether or not the organization is a good fit for you.

· · · ● · ● · ● · ·

## Thriving in the Workplace

Coping with workplace stress and expectations

There I was, in the fast-paced world of television, switching between on-screen and off-screen roles. To anyone looking in, I must have seemed like the consummate extrovert: lively, upbeat, and always in the thick of things. They had no idea that I was actually an introvert who was having trouble reconciling my shyness with the demands of my job.

In my role as a TV host, I was expected to maintain a level of enthusiasm and audience interaction that didn't always come easily to me. But when the lights went out, I often felt depleted and longed for some solitude in which to refuel. My work in the background also required me to put on a mask of extroversion and interact with others outside of my comfort zone.

The hardest part was learning to interact with clients, go to networking events, and understand the culture of my field. One event, in particular, was draining because I had to pretend to be friendly and outgoing with a large number of strangers. It was like putting on a performance, and all I wanted to do was find a place to myself where I could rest and recover from the ordeal.

The longer I pretended to be outgoing, the more I realized that it was damaging my mental and emotional health. Because of the demands of my job in television, I had to figure out how to be both an introvert and an extrovert. In response, I began establishing personal limits, such as going to fewer gatherings and making more time for reflection and relaxation. I also started recognizing and appreciating my introverted strengths, such as my attentiveness and ability to observe and learn about others.

Slowly but surely, I learned to navigate the television industry while staying true to my introverted self. I learned that I can be successful in a high-stress profession without compromising my own needs and happiness. It took some trial and error, but I was able to find the equilibrium between the demands of my career and my need for solitude.

Welcome to the workplace, where I/HSPs can feel like square pegs in round holes!

Navigating the complexities of the workplace, coping with stress, and meeting expectations can be challenging for anyone, but I/HSPs often face unique obstacles due to their natural tendencies and sensitivities. But with the right strategies and way of thinking, it's possible for an introvert or HSP to not only get by at work but also to do well.

In this section, we'll talk about the problems that I/HSPs may face at work, such as managing stress, dealing with sensory overload, and adjusting to a world that often values extroverted traits. We will also talk about tips and plans for overcoming these problems and making the most of your unique strengths and skills.

By learning about the needs and preferences of I/HSPs, you can learn to deal with stress and expectations at work better, which will help you do well in your chosen career path. As an introvert or HSP, your ability to empathize, think deeply, and stay focused can be very useful at work. By being aware of these strengths and learning to speak up for yourself, you can build a successful and fulfilling career.

So, let's talk about how you can learn to be proud of your unique qualities and feel confident in the workplace.

**To deal with stress and expectations, try the following:**

1. **Establish boundaries:** Set limits on your time and energy by setting up regular breaks and telling your coworkers and bosses what you need.

2. **Prioritize tasks:** Focus on getting the most important things done first, and if you can, try not to do more than one thing at a time.

3. **Develop a support network:** Build relationships with coworkers who can understand your needs and help you out.

4. **Practice self-care:** Make sure you take care of your physical and mental health outside of work by eating well, getting enough sleep, and exercising.

· · · ● · ● · ● · ·

## Networking and building professional relationships

Networking can be scary for people who are shy or highly sensitive. It frequently evokes images of crowded rooms, shallow conversations, and the pressure to make a lasting impression. However, networking and developing professional relationships are essential to career success, and it is entirely possible for I/HSPs to approach networking in a genuine and effective manner.

The unique qualities of I/HSPs can be used to great advantage in the workplace.

They can become powerful networkers by making use of their innate sympathy, attentiveness, and ability to form meaningful connections with others.

If you're an introvert or highly sensitive person looking to network and build professional relationships, consider the following advice:

1. **Embrace quality over quantity:** Instead of trying to meet everyone at an event, focus on making a few strong connections. Deep, genuine connections are more valuable than a long list of superficial acquaintances.

2. **Leverage your listening skills:** Because of their exceptional listening skills, I/HSPs can make excellent networkers. To demonstrate that you are interested in the other person, make an effort to listen carefully and ask probing questions.

3. **Find smaller, more intimate networking events:** You can have more meaningful conversations at smaller events or industry-specific meetups than at large, impersonal gatherings.

4. **Prepare conversation topics:** Prepare a list of engaging questions or points of discussion. This can make small talk less of an ordeal and open the door to more meaningful exchanges with others.

5. **Use online networking:** I/HSPs can benefit from using social media platforms and online forums to connect with professionals in their field. Participate in

online discussions, share your work, and connect with people whose work you admire.

6. **Practice self-care:** Networking can be exhausting for I/HSPs, so prioritize self-care. Allow yourself to take breaks and recharge during events, and make sure you have downtime planned afterward.

7. **Follow up and nurture relationships:** After meeting someone new, send a personalized message expressing your appreciation for the conversation and your desire to stay in touch. Maintain contact and nurture these relationships over time by sharing relevant articles and offering assistance as needed.

8. **Be authentic:** When networking, embrace your individuality and be yourself. If you're genuine, you'll be liked by more people and have deeper connections with them.

If you follow these guidelines, networking will no longer be something you dread doing, but rather something you can use to your advantage and boost your career. Keep in mind that collecting business cards isn't the end goal; making genuine connections is. With effort and time, you can build a network of contacts who will cheer you on as you climb the professional ladder and encourage your own development.

## Asserting yourself and advocating for your needs

It's important for an introvert or HSP to speak up for themselves and make sure their needs are met on the job. This can make it more likely that you'll get the help and adjustments you need to succeed. Think about these suggestions:

- **Be proactive:** Put your needs out there before they become a problem. For example, you could ask for a more peaceful work environment, altered working hours, or specialized assistance with a particular project.

- **Practice effective communication:** Express your wants and needs eloquently while remaining polite and assertive. Don't come across as passive-aggressive or overly emotional.

- **Find allies:** Find coworkers or superiors who will listen to your concerns and help you advocate for yourself.

. . . . •. • •. . .

## Career Advancement

Setting and achieving professional goals

Setting and achieving career goals that are in line with your passions and interests is essential as you advance in your chosen field. Remember these pointers:

- **Set SMART goals:** Create specific, measurable, achievable, relevant, and time-bound goals to help you stay focused and motivated.

- **Create an action plan:** Break your goals down into smaller, manageable steps and develop a timeline for achieving each step.

- **Track your progress:** Regularly evaluate your progress and adjust your goals or action plan as needed.

- **Celebrate your accomplishments:** As you work toward your objectives, take time to appreciate and celebrate your progress, no matter how small.

. . . •. • • . . .

## Navigating Promotions and Job Transitions: A Roller Coaster Ride for I/HSPs

Promotions and changing jobs, a familiar topic.

For I/HSPs, they can be like an exhilarating roller coaster ride, complete with ups, downs, twists, turns, and the occasional scream (hopefully not in the workplace). As thrilling as the ride may be, it can also be challenging to navigate these changes in a way that doesn't leave you feeling queasy at the end.

If you're an introvert or highly sensitive person, here's how to handle a promotion or job change with grace:

1. **Unleash your inner detective:** Before accepting a promotion or transitioning to a new job, do some sleuthing. Research the role, its responsibilities, and maybe even the office gossip (within reason, of course) to ensure it aligns with your strengths and interests. You wouldn't buy a new car without checking its specs, right? Apply the same principle to your career moves.

2. **Assemble your career Avengers:** Reach out to colleagues or mentors who have experience in the new role for advice and support. They'll be like your personal superheroes, swooping in with valuable insights and pep talks when you need them most.

3. **Channel your inner chameleon:** Be adaptable and embrace change with open arms (or at least a firm handshake). Remember that it's normal to feel like a fish out of water at first. But just like a chameleon, you'll soon adapt to your new surroundings, blend in, and maybe even learn some sweet new skills.

4. **Find your Zen:** As you take on additional responsibilities, ensure you're maintaining a healthy balance between your work and personal life. Practice the ancient art of "not bringing work home" and set aside time for relaxation, hobbies, and self-care. You can't conquer the corporate world if you're running on empty.

5. **Celebrate your victories:** Whether it's successfully leading your first meeting or finally figuring out how to use that fancy new coffee machine in the break room, take a moment to acknowledge your accomplishments. It's all part of the roller coaster ride, and you deserve to enjoy the view from the top.

6. **Bring your sense of humor:** Last but not least, don't let the ups and downs of promotions and job changes dampen your sense of humor. You'll be better

prepared to deal with difficulties if you can laugh at yourself, even in the face of adversity.

So, enjoy the ups and downs of getting new jobs and getting promoted. If you can maintain your sense of humor, remain flexible, and lean on those around you for support, you'll not only make it through this ordeal unscathed, but you might even emerge from it with a greater appreciation for your own strength.

· · · · ● · ● · · ·

## Developing Leadership Skills: How I/HSPs Can Rule the World (or at Least the Office)

Whoever said that I/HSPs can't be great leaders was clearly wrong. In fact, I/HSPs can make great leaders if they know how to succeed in their unique styles.

In fact, the following are examples of well-known leaders who are also introverts or highly sensitive people:

- The Indian independence leader **Mahatma Gandhi** was known for his reserved and reflective nature. He once said, "In a gentle way, you can shake the world."

- It has been said that **Abraham Lincoln**, the 16th President of the United States, was a man of few words. He was also known for his empathy and emotional intelligence.

- **Eleanor Roosevelt**, the former First Lady and human rights activist was said to be an introvert. She used her quiet strength and intelligence to speak up for people and groups that didn't have a lot of power.

- **Rosa Parks** was a civil rights activist who refused to give up her seat on a bus in Montgomery, Alabama. She was also described as an introvert. Her quiet act of defiance started a movement.

- **Emma Watson,** the actress and activist has identified as both an introvert and an

HSP. She has spoken about the importance of self-care and setting boundaries.

- **Barack Obama** has been described as introverted. He is known for his calm and measured demeanor, and his ability to connect with people on a deeper level.

- **Bill Gates**, co-founder of Microsoft and philanthropist has been described as introverted. He has spoken about the importance of taking time for oneself and disconnecting from technology.

- **Albert Einstein**, the famous physicist was known for his quiet and introspective nature. He once said, "The monotony and solitude of a quiet life stimulates the creative mind."

- **Princess Diana** was described as both an introvert and an empath. She used her platform to advocate for social causes and connect with people on a personal level.

So, let's dive into the world of leadership development for I/HSPs:

1. **Become a superhero:** Leverage your innate abilities, such as active listening, empathy, and thoughtful decision-making, to lead and inspire others. Think of yourself as the quiet superhero of the office, using your powers for good and occasionally swooping in to save the day.

2. **Build your workplace "family":** Foster meaningful connections with your team members by showing genuine interest in their lives and work. You'll be like the cool aunt or uncle at family gatherings, creating a bond that goes beyond the 9-to-5 grind.

3. **Embrace your inner Oprah:** Encourage collaboration and create an inclusive environment where everyone feels heard and valued. Channel your inner talk show host and make sure everyone has a seat at the table, figuratively speaking (unless you actually have a really big table).

4. **Cultivate a feedback garden:** Regularly seek feedback from your team and be open to constructive criticism. Think of it as planting seeds for personal growth and improvement. Sure, some seeds might be a little prickly, but with the right care and attention, you'll soon be harvesting a bountiful crop of leadership skills.

5. **Master the art of delegation:** As an introvert or HSP, you might be tempted to take on every task yourself. But a great leader knows how to delegate effectively. So, practice the ancient art of "You Do It" and entrust your team with responsibilities that play to their strengths.

6. **Become a motivational speaker (in your own way):** You don't have to be Tony Robbins to inspire your team. Use your quiet charisma and thoughtful communication style to motivate and encourage others. Remember, a well-timed, genuine compliment can go a long way.

7. Celebrate victories with style: Whether it's a major project milestone or simply making it through a particularly rough Monday, find creative ways to celebrate your team's achievements. This could involve anything from a heartfelt email to an impromptu office dance party (with a designated quiet corner for I/HSPs, of course).

Successfully navigating the challenges of adulting in the workplace requires an understanding of your unique strengths and needs as an introvert or HSP. Accept who you really are, wrap yourself in a leadership cape made of imagination, and fly through life. Who knows? You might just change the world—or at the very least, create a more harmonious and productive office environment.

# CHAPTER FOUR

## FINANCIAL ADULTING

### Budgeting and Saving

CREATING A REALISTIC BUDGET

As an introvert or HSP, you might be great at putting your books in alphabetical order, but let's be honest: not everyone is a financial genius. This is where making a budget that makes sense comes in. Trust me, you don't have to be a millionaire on Wall Street to handle your money well.

Although there has been research into the correlation between character traits and economic decisions, there is less data comparing the wealth of introverts/HSPs and extroverts.

Overall, it is difficult to draw definitive conclusions about the relationship between introversion/HSP and financial health based on the available research. It's possible that people's personalities influence how they handle money, but it's also likely that many other factors (including income, education, and life circumstances) play a role.

With that in mind, consider the following suggestions for trimming costs and balancing your budget:

1. **Track your income and expenses:** Write down all your income sources and

how much you spend each month. You can use an app or go old school with pen and paper (bonus points if you use a quill).

2. **Categorize your expenses:** Divide your expenses into essential (rent, groceries, bills) and non-essential (that artisanal coffee you can't resist). Remember, even introverts need some fun money for those cozy nights in.

3. **Set spending limits:** Determine how much you're willing to spend in each category. Be realistic, and don't be too hard on yourself – we all need that occasional treat to recharge our introvert batteries.

· · · · ●·●· · ·

## Saving money and establishing an emergency fund

The introvert's guide to saving money should include a chapter on hibernation. Unfortunately, we can't all be bears, so we'll have to save money the old-fashioned way:

- **Automate your savings:** Set up an automatic transfer from your checking to your savings account each month. Out of sight, out of mind, right?

- **Cut back on non-essentials:** Re-evaluate your expenses and see where you can cut back. Maybe it's time to embrace the art of cooking and ditch the takeout? You'll save money and become the introvert Martha Stewart.

- Establish an emergency fund: Aim to save at least 3-6 months' worth of living expenses. You never know when life will throw a curveball, like a surprise invitation to a social event you can't avoid.

· · · ●·●· · · ·

## Managing debt and loans

The path to financial independence isn't always smooth, but that shouldn't discourage you. Here's how an introvert ninja would attack credit card debt:

1. **Make a debt repayment plan:** List your debts, interest rates, and minimum payments. Prioritize them and decide how much extra you can pay each month.

2. **Consider the debt snowball or avalanche method:** The snowball method involves paying off the smallest debt first, while the avalanche method focuses on the highest interest rate. Choose the one that appeals to your inner introvert strategist.

3. **Refinance or consolidate loans:** Look into refinancing or consolidating your loans to get better terms or lower interest rates. Just make sure to do your research to avoid any hidden traps or unnecessary social interactions.

• • • ● • ● • • •

## Investing and Planning for the Future

Making smart financial decisions

Who says managing money can't be fun and engaging? It's time to put on our financial adulting hats, embrace our inner Warren Buffett, and dive into the world of smart decision-making. In this section, I'll provide you with the knowledge and tools you need to set achievable financial goals, create a realistic financial timeline, and find the right advisor who can guide you through the complexities of money management. So let's get started, fellow I/HSPs, and prove that we're more than capable of making informed financial decisions that can positively impact our lives.

- **Set financial goals:** Whether it's saving for a down payment on a house or treating yourself to a solo vacation, establish clear financial goals and work towards them.

- **Create a financial timeline:** Consider your short-term and long-term financial plans. Break them down into achievable steps and remember to celebrate your successes along the way.

- **Consult a financial advisor:** If the thought of managing your finances makes you want to curl up in a blanket fort, consider seeking professional advice.

• • • ● • ● • • •

## Building a retirement plan

Retirement might seem far away, but it's never too early to start planning for those golden years of introverted bliss. Here's how to build a retirement plan that'll have you sipping tea in your dream cottage:

1. **Calculate your retirement needs:** Estimate how much money you'll need to maintain your desired lifestyle in retirement. Don't forget to factor in your hobbies and interests.

2. **Maximize your retirement savings:** Contribute to your employer-sponsored retirement plan, like a 401(k) or an IRA. If your employer offers matching contributions, make sure to take full advantage of it – it's basically free money!

3. **Diversify your investments:** As the old saying goes, "Don't put all your eggs in one basket." Spread your investments across various assets to minimize risks and maximize returns.

• • • ● • ● • • •

## Investing in stocks, bonds, and other financial assets

Investing can seem like an intimidating maze to navigate, but don't let that stop you. You, too, can become a smart investor with the right help and a little bit of patience. Here, we'll break down the basics of investing so that even novices can make informed decisions and have fun with the process.

**Starting small: Low-cost index funds and ETFs**

For beginners or those looking to dip their toes into the investment pool, low-cost index funds and exchange-traded funds (ETFs) are a great starting point. These investment vehicles offer several advantages, such as:

- **Diversification:** Diversifying your portfolio helps protect your assets from the potential collapse of any single holding.

- **Low fees:** Index funds and ETFs typically have lower fees compared to actively managed funds, which means more of your money goes towards building your investment portfolio.

- **Easy to buy and sell:** You can buy and sell ETFs just like stocks, giving you flexibility and control over your investments.

· · · ● · ● · · ·

## Educating Yourself: Resources for the introverted investor

Knowledge is power, especially when it comes to investing. Fortunately, there's a wealth of resources available for I/HSPs who prefer learning at their own pace:

- **Books:**
  There are many books available for investors of all skill levels, from novices to seasoned pros.

For those just starting out in the investment world, I recommend the following books:

1. "The Little Book of Common Sense Investing" by John C. Bogle - This book offers simple, practical advice on low-cost, long-term investing using index funds.

2. "Rich Dad Poor Dad" by Robert Kiyosaki - A classic personal finance book that emphasizes the importance of financial education and building wealth through investments.

3. "The Simple Path to Wealth" by J.L. Collins - This book provides a straightforward guide to investing in low-cost index funds and achieving financial independence.

4. "The Bogleheads' Guide to Investing" by Taylor Larimore, Mel Lindauer, and Michael LeBoeuf - Based on the investing philosophy of John Bogle, this book offers a step-by-step guide to creating a diversified investment portfolio.

5. "The Millionaire Next Door" by Thomas J. Stanley and William D. Danko - This book offers insights into the habits and characteristics of wealthy individuals, focusing on the importance of living below your means and investing wisely.

6. "The Richest Man in Babylon" by George S. Clason - Through parables set in ancient Babylon, this book imparts timeless wisdom on managing personal finances and investing for the future.

7. "One Up on Wall Street" by Peter Lynch - Written by a legendary investor, this book teaches beginners how to analyze stocks and find promising investment opportunities.

- **Online courses:**
  Websites like Coursera and Udemy offer a wide range of investing courses, covering topics from the basics to more specialized areas like options trading or cryptocurrency.

- **Podcasts:**
  Listen to investing podcasts while you're on the go, such as "The Indicator from Planet Money" or "InvestED."

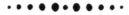

## Developing your investment strategy

Now that you know the fundamentals of investing, you can work on creating a plan that is tailored to your specific needs. Here are a few things to keep in mind:

- **Risk tolerance:** As an introvert or HSP, you might prefer a more conservative approach to investing. Determine your risk tolerance and choose investments that align with your comfort level.

- **Time horizon:** Consider how long you plan to invest before needing to access your funds. Longer time horizons typically allow for more aggressive investment strategies, while shorter time horizons call for a more conservative approach.

- **Asset allocation:** Allocate your investments across various asset classes (stocks, bonds, real estate, etc.) to minimize risk and optimize returns.

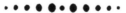

## Staying the course: Patience and discipline

Investing is a long game, so it's important to stay the course regardless of temporary ups and downs in the market. Remember, slow and steady wins the race, especially for I/HSPs. Here are a few tips to help you stay the course:

- **Review your investments periodically:** Regularly assess your portfolio to ensure it's still aligned with your financial goals and risk tolerance. Make adjustments as needed, but avoid excessive trading or knee-jerk reactions to market events.

- **Reinvest dividends:** Reinvesting dividends can help grow your investment portfolio faster by taking advantage of compounding returns.

- Keep emotions in check: It's natural to feel anxious or worried during market downturns, but resist the urge to make impulsive decisions based on emotions. Stick to your investment plan and focus on the long-term outlook.

Follow these comprehensive guidelines and embrace your unique strengths as an introvert or HSP, and you will successfully navigate the world of investing and build a secure financial future.

· · · · • · • · · ·

## Navigating Financial Challenges

### Handling unexpected expenses

Life has a funny way of throwing us curveballs when we least expect them. Here's how to deal with unexpected expenses without losing your cool (or your budget):

1. **Build an emergency fund:** I can't stress this enough. Having an emergency fund will save you from going into debt when unexpected expenses arise.

2. **Assess your options:** If you can't cover the expense with your emergency fund, explore other options like a personal loan or a balance transfer credit card with a low-interest rate.

3. **Revisit your budget:** Adjust your budget to accommodate the unexpected expense. This might mean cutting back on non-essential spending for a while, but your future self will thank you.

· · · · • · • · · ·

## Recovering from financial setbacks

Even the most financially responsible people can face setbacks. Here's how to bounce back and regain your financial footing:

- **Don't be too hard on yourself:** Remember, everyone faces financial challenges at some point. Cut yourself some slack and focus on finding a solution.

- **Create a plan:** Identify the root cause of the setback and develop a plan to address it. This might involve adjusting your budget, increasing your income, or seeking professional help.

- **Stay accountable:** Share your financial goals with a trusted friend or family member who can offer support and encouragement along the way.

• • • • • • • • • •

## Planning for major life events

From weddings to buying a home, major life events can be expensive. Here's how to plan for them without breaking the bank (or your introvert spirit):

- **Start saving early:** As soon as you know a major life event is on the horizon, start saving. The earlier you begin, the more time you have to reach your financial goals.

- **Set a realistic budget:** Determine how much you can realistically afford to spend on the event without going into debt.

- **Get creative:** Find ways to save money without sacrificing the experience. For example, a small, intimate wedding might be more appealing to an introvert than an extravagant affair.

• • • • • • • • • •

## Embracing frugality and minimalism

I/HSPs often find value in simplicity. By embracing frugality and minimalism, you can reduce financial stress and focus on what truly matters:

1. **Practice mindful spending:** Before making a purchase, ask yourself if it's necessary and if it will truly add value to your life. This can help you avoid impulse buys and save money in the long run.

2. **Declutter your possessions:** Take time to assess what you own and let go of items that no longer serve a purpose. You might even make some extra cash by selling unwanted items.

3. **Focus on experiences over possessions:** Invest in experiences that align with your introverted and highly sensitive nature, such as solo trips, personal development, or hobbies that bring joy and fulfillment.

Financial adulting does not have to be a daunting task for I/HSPs. You can handle your personal finances with confidence and grace if you follow these suggestions and play to your strengths.

It's not about being perfect, but about developing sound money management practices that complement your reserved and perceptive way of life.

# CHAPTER FIVE

## SELF-CARE AND PERSONAL GROWTH

I N THIS CHAPTER, WE'LL explore the world of self-care and personal growth, specifically tailored to the unique needs of I/HSPs. If you're an introvert or a highly sensitive person, the fast-paced, noisy world around you might make you feel overwhelmed. To do well in this kind of setting, you need to take care of yourself physically and mentally. Self-care and personal growth aren't just nice things to do for yourself; they're important parts of a well-balanced, happy life.

Self-care and personal development look different for I/HSPs than they do for their extroverted peers. For example, I/HSPs often need more downtime to get their energy back and figure out how they feel. This means that they may need to focus more on quiet, introspective activities that help them think and relax as a way to take care of themselves.

Another big difference is that I/HSPs may be more sensitive to things like bright lights, loud noises, and strong emotions. This increased sensitivity can make some self-care activities, like working out hard or going to a big party, feel overwhelming. In this chapter, we'll talk about ways to take care of yourself that meet the special needs of I/HSPs. This will help you move through the world with more ease and confidence.

We'll also talk about personal growth, which is important for introverts, HSPs, and extroverts alike. Even though I/HSPs may develop themselves in different ways, they are both still able to reach their goals and reach their full potential. In fact, their tendency to think a lot about themselves and their ability to observe things well can help them grow as people.

Physical, mental, and emotional health are just some of the aspects of self-care and development that we'll explore in this chapter. We will also provide resources to help you develop routines and habits that cater to your specific needs as an introvert or HSP. In other words, you're about to embark on an insightful quest of self-discovery that's designed with the unique strengths of I/HSPs in mind.

· • • ● • ● • • ·

## Physical Well-being

### The Mind-Body Connection

As I/HSPs, we're all about our inner world, but it's essential not to neglect our physical health. Research shows a strong connection between physical health and mental health, with one positively (or negatively) impacting the other[1] . So let's dive into the world of physical well-being!

## Sleep: Your Secret Weapon

We all know that sleep is important, but it's especially crucial for I/HSPs. Sleep helps us recharge our introvert batteries and process the stimuli we've encountered during the day[2] . Here are some tips for getting quality sleep:

1. **Create a consistent sleep schedule:** Going to bed and waking up at the same

---

1. Warburton, D. E., Nicol, C. W., & Bredin, S. S. (2006). Health benefits of physical activity: the evidence. Canadian medical association journal, 174(6), 801-809. https://pubmed.ncbi.nlm.nih.gov/16534088/

time every day helps regulate your internal clock.

2. **Develop a bedtime routine:** Engage in calming activities before bed, like reading, journaling, or taking a warm bath.

3. **Limit screen time before bed:** The blue light emitted by screens can mess with our sleep hormones, so try to unplug at least an hour before bedtime.

4. **Optimize your sleep environment:** Make sure your bedroom is cool, dark, and quiet. You can use blackout curtains, earplugs, or a white noise machine to help create a sleep-friendly atmosphere.

5. **Choose the right mattress and pillow:** Invest in a comfortable, supportive mattress and pillow that cater to your preferred sleeping position and provide proper spinal alignment.

6. **Avoid caffeine and alcohol close to bedtime:** Both substances can interfere with your sleep cycle. Try to avoid consuming them at least 4-6 hours before bedtime.

7. **Practice relaxation techniques:** Deep breathing exercises, progressive muscle relaxation, or guided imagery can help calm your mind and prepare your body for sleep.

8. **Get regular physical activity:** Engaging in daily exercise can help improve your sleep quality, but try to avoid intense workouts close to bedtime as they may leave you feeling too energized to sleep.

9. **Be mindful of your diet:** Eating a heavy meal right before bedtime can cause discomfort and make it difficult to fall asleep. Instead, opt for a light, nutritious snack if you're hungry before bed.

10. **Manage stress:** Developing healthy stress-management techniques, such as practicing yoga or meditation, can help you unwind and sleep better.

11. **Limit daytime naps:** While napping can be beneficial, excessive or poorly timed naps can disrupt your nighttime sleep. Keep naps short (20-30 minutes) and avoid napping too close to bedtime.

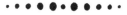

## A Clean Space = A Clear Mind

A cluttered space can lead to a cluttered mind, so maintaining a clean and organized living environment can help you feel more at ease. Plus, tidying up can be a form of self-care, giving you a sense of accomplishment and control[3]. The benefits of a clean and organized space extend beyond aesthetics; they can have a profound impact on your mental health, productivity, and overall well-being.

To create a harmonious living space that supports your introverted or highly sensitive nature, consider the following tips:

1. **Create designated areas for specific activities:** Allocate specific areas in your home for work, relaxation, and hobbies. This will help you mentally separate these different aspects of your life, making it easier to focus and unwind when needed.

2. **Establish a decluttering routine:** Regularly decluttering your space can prevent the buildup of clutter and make it easier to maintain a clean environment. Set aside time each week or month to go through your belongings and decide what to keep, donate, or discard.

3. **Optimize storage solutions:** Invest in functional storage solutions that help you keep your belongings organized and easily accessible. This can include shelves, drawers, and storage boxes that allow you to store items neatly and efficiently.

4. **Create a calming atmosphere:** Use soft lighting, calming colors, and soothing scents to make your space feel more inviting and relaxing. Consider adding plants, artwork, or other personal touches that bring you joy and create a sense

3. Saxbe, D. E., & Repetti, R. L. (2010). No place like home: Home tours correlate with daily patterns of mood and cortisol. Personality and Social Psychology Bulletin, 36(1), 71-81. https://pubmed.ncbi.nlm.nih.gov/19934011/

of serenity.

5. **Prioritize cleanliness:** Set a cleaning schedule to ensure that your living space remains clean and hygienic. Regularly vacuum, dust, and wipe down surfaces to keep your environment fresh and healthy.

6. **Break tasks into manageable chunks:** Cleaning and organizing can feel overwhelming, especially for I/HSPs who may be more sensitive to the chaos. Break tasks into smaller, manageable steps and tackle them one at a time to make the process more enjoyable.

7. **Practice gratitude for your space:** Acknowledge and appreciate the comfort, safety, and functionality your living space provides. Cultivating gratitude can make it easier to maintain a clean and organized environment.

· · · ● ● · ● · · ·

## Exercise: Not Just for Gym Rats

Exercise is essential for mental health, as it releases endorphins that help reduce stress and improve mood[4]. As I/HSPs, we might not be into high-intensity workouts or group fitness classes, but there are plenty of low-impact exercise options:

- **Yoga:** A gentle way to build strength, flexibility, and mindfulness.

- **Pilates:** A low-impact workout that focuses on core strength and body alignment.

- **Walking:** A simple yet effective way to get moving and connect with nature.

---

4. Peluso, M. A., & Guerra de Andrade, L. H. (2005). Physical activity and mental health: the association between exercise and mood. Clinics, 60(1), 61-70. https://pubmed.ncbi.nlm.nih.gov/15838583/

• • • •**•**•**•**• • •

## Nourishing Your Body: Food as Fuel

Eating well is a critical aspect of self-care. It's not just about counting calories or following fad diets; it's about nourishing your body with whole foods and balanced nutrition. Here are some tips:

- **Meal planning and preparation:** Set aside time each week to plan and prepare meals, making it easier to eat well throughout the week.

- **Whole foods and balanced nutrition:** Prioritize whole, unprocessed foods, and make sure your meals include a mix of protein, healthy fats, and complex carbohydrates.

- **Avoid emotional eating:** As HSPs, we might be prone to emotional eating[5]. Recognize your triggers and find healthier ways to cope with emotions.

• • • •**•**•**•**• • •

## Mental Health and Emotional Well-being

### The Unique Mental Health Landscape of I/HSPs

I/HSPs may face unique mental health challenges due to our sensitivity to stimuli and need for solitude. I've got some strategies to help you maintain your mental health and emotional well-being.

---

5. Arnow, B., Kenardy, J., & Agras, W. S. (1995). The Emotional Eating Scale: The development of a measure to assess coping with negative affect by eating. International Journal of Eating Disorders, 18(1), 79-90. https://pubmed.ncbi.nlm.nih.gov/7670446/

**Mindfulness and Meditation: Your Mental Health BFFs**

Mindfulness and meditation have been shown to help reduce stress, improve focus, and increase overall well-being[6] . Here are some tips to incorporate these practices into your daily life:

1. **Start small and be consistent:** Begin with just a few minutes of meditation each day, gradually increasing the duration as you become more comfortable. Consistency is more important than the length of each session.

2. **Create a dedicated meditation space:** Set up a quiet, comfortable space where you can practice meditation without distractions. This can be a corner of your room, a specific chair, or even a spot in your garden.

3. **Find a practice that works for you:** With so many meditation styles available, it's essential to find one that resonates with you and fits your needs. Experiment with different techniques and resources until you find the one that feels most natural and enjoyable. Meditation comes in many different styles, allowing you to find the one that resonates with you the most. Some popular meditation styles include:

- **Mindfulness meditation:** This practice involves focusing on your breath and bringing your attention back to it whenever your mind wanders. It teaches you to be present and aware of your thoughts and emotions without judgment.

- **Loving-kindness meditation (Metta):** This type of meditation cultivates feelings of love, kindness, and compassion for yourself and others. It involves silently repeating positive phrases or affirmations, such as "May I be happy, may I be healthy, may I be safe."

- **Body scan meditation:** This practice involves systematically scanning your body from head to toe, focusing on each body part, and releasing any tension

---

6. Goyal, M., Singh, S., Sibinga, E. M., Gould, N. F., Rowland-Seymour, A., Sharma, R., ... & Haythornthwaite, J. A. (2014). Meditation programs for psychological stress and well-being: a systematic review and meta-analysis. JAMA Internal Medicine, 174(3), 357-368. https://pubmed.ncbi.nlm.nih.gov/24395196/

or discomfort you might notice.

- **Guided meditation:** Guided meditation involves listening to a recorded meditation or following along with a meditation app, where an instructor guides you through the practice step by step.

- **Transcendental Meditation (TM):** TM is a specific technique that involves the repetition of a personal mantra given to you by a certified TM teacher. It's typically practiced for 20 minutes twice a day.

- **Walking meditation:** Walking meditation combines mindfulness with gentle movement. As you walk slowly and deliberately, focus on the sensations in your body and the rhythm of your breath.

• • • ● • ● • • •

## Managing Stress and Anxiety

As I/HSPs, we may be more susceptible to stress and anxiety due to our sensitivity to stimuli and need for downtime[7] . Here are some coping strategies:

- **Identify sources of stress and anxiety:** Understanding what triggers your stress and anxiety can help you develop effective coping strategies.

- **Seek professional help:** Therapy and counseling can be beneficial for managing stress and anxiety, especially if you find it difficult to cope on your own.

- **Practice self-compassion:** Remember that it's okay to need downtime and solitude. Be kind to yourself and prioritize your well-being.

---

7. Grillon, C., Robinson, O. J., Mathur, A., & Ernst, M. (2016). Effect of attention control on sustained attention during induced anxiety. Cognition and Emotion, 30(4), 700-712. https://psycnet.apa.org/record/2016-13771-008

Practicing self-compassion is essential for introverts and HSP's, as it helps you acknowledge and accept your unique needs without judgment. By cultivating self-compassion, you give yourself permission to prioritize your well-being and make choices that support your emotional health.

One way to practice self-compassion is to recognize your self-critical thoughts. Pay attention to your inner dialogue and notice when you're being harsh or judgmental towards yourself. Acknowledge these thoughts and remind yourself that it's okay to need downtime and solitude.

Another approach is to replace self-criticism with self-kindness. When you notice self-critical thoughts, take a moment to pause and consider how you would respond to a friend in a similar situation. Offer yourself the same understanding, encouragement, and support that you would extend to someone you care about.

It's also important to practice mindfulness as part of self-compassion. This means being aware of your thoughts, feelings, and bodily sensations without judgment or resistance. One way to develop self-love and acceptance is to practice mindfulness and live in the moment.

It's okay to stop what you're doing and rest whenever you need to. People who are introverted or highly sensitive may need more time alone to recharge. You should not feel bad or selfish for satisfying these desires. In addition to the obvious health benefits, prioritizing your own well-being also allows you to be your most effective self in other contexts.

Lastly, consider developing a self-compassion mantra or affirmation that you can use during moments of self-doubt or criticism. This could be a simple phrase like, "I am enough," or "I am worthy of love and care." Repeating this mantra can help you cultivate a more compassionate relationship with yourself and remind you of your inherent worth.

• • • ● • ● • • •

## Building Resilience and Coping Skills

Developing resilience is essential for navigating life's ups and downs. Here are some strategies for building resilience and coping skills:

- **Embrace a growth mindset:** View setbacks as opportunities for growth and learning, rather than failures.

- **Develop a strong support network:** Surround yourself with people who understand and support your needs as an introvert or HSP.

• • • ● • ● • • ·

## Personal Development

Personal development is an ongoing journey of self-improvement and growth. As I/HSPs, we can benefit from setting goals, cultivating habits, and embracing lifelong learning.

### Setting Personal Goals

Goal-setting can help you stay focused and motivated on your personal development journey. Here are some tips for setting achievable goals:

- **Be specific and realistic:** Break down your goals into smaller, manageable steps.

- **Set deadlines:** Give yourself a timeframe for achieving your goals to maintain motivation.

- **Track your progress:** Regularly assess your progress and adjust your goals as needed.

· · · · ● · ● · · ·

## Cultivating Habits for Success

Our habits shape our lives and determine our success. Here are some tips for creating and maintaining healthy habits:

- **Start small:** Focus on one habit at a time and gradually build upon your successes.

- **Establish routines:** Incorporate your new habits into your daily routine for consistency.

- **Be patient:** Remember that it takes time to break old habits and create new ones.

· · · · ● · ● · · ·

## Embracing Lifelong Learning

Lifelong learning is an essential aspect of personal development, helping you stay engaged, curious, and adaptable. Here are some strategies for incorporating learning into daily life:

- **Read:** Books, articles, and blogs are excellent resources for expanding your knowledge.

- **Take courses:** Online courses, workshops, and seminars can help you develop new skills and explore new interests.

- **Join groups:** Connect with like-minded individuals who share your passion for learning and personal growth.

I/HSPs can lead happy, healthy lives if they take care of their bodies and minds. As you continue on your path to "adulting," don't forget to put yourself first, show yourself compassion, and commit to growing as a person.

# CHAPTER SIX

# HOBBIES AND LEISURE ACTIVITIES FOR I/HSPs

WELCOME TO THE WONDROUS world of hobbies, where introverts and HSP's can thrive and flourish! In this chapter, we'll dive deep into various hobbies and leisure activities that cater to your unique personality traits. You'll be able to explore the realms of creativity, socialization, self-improvement, and more. And of course, we'll sprinkle in some humor and wit along the way because, let's face it, adulting is hard, but finding hobbies shouldn't be.

## Creative Pursuits

**Exploring your passions and interests.**

- Make a list of your interests, and don't be shy about it! From knitting cat sweaters to assembling intricate ship models, there's no judgment here.

- Take a stroll through an arts and crafts store, or better yet, Pinterest! Let your imagination run wild and see what catches your eye.

- Give yourself permission to try new things. Remember, Picasso wasn't born with a paintbrush in his hand. Well, maybe he was, but you get the point.

**Finding joy in solitude and quiet**

- Embrace the silence! When there is nothing but your own thoughts around you, creative activities like painting, drawing, or writing can be therapeutic.

- Try "quiet" hobbies like calligraphy, adult coloring, or assembling jigsaw puzzles. They're like a mini-meditation session without the actual meditation.

- Create a peaceful space in your home dedicated to your hobbies. If you can't have a whole room, just find a cozy corner.

**Cultivating a creative and fulfilling life**

- Allow yourself the freedom to experiment and make mistakes. Your first masterpiece might just be a gloriously terrible stick figure.

- Set aside regular time to engage in your creative pursuits. Even if it's just 15 minutes a day, consistency is key.

- Share your creations with friends and family, or keep them secret like a modern-day Banksy. Either way, you're still awesome.

• • • • ● • ● • • •

# Social Hobbies

Engaging in group activities that suit your personality

- Look for activities with a smaller, more intimate group size. Think book clubs, not 300-person flash mobs.

- Seek out activities that allow for breaks or quiet moments, like board game nights, where you can recharge your social batteries.

- Consider joining a group that revolves around a shared interest, like photography or knitting. It's easier to connect with people when you have something in common.

**Building connections through shared interests**

- Remember that it's okay to be an introvert in a social setting. You don't have to be the life of the party to make meaningful connections.

- Be open to meeting new people, but don't feel pressured to become instant BFFs with everyone you meet. Quality over quantity!

- Share your experiences with others in online forums or social media groups, where you can connect with like-minded individuals without the overwhelm of face-to-face interactions.

**Tips for joining clubs and organizations**

- Research clubs and organizations in your area that align with your interests. It's like online dating, but for hobbies.

- Attend a few events or meetings as a guest to get a feel for the group dynamics before committing to membership.

- Be prepared for a bit of small talk, but remember, it's just the appetizer before the main course of awesome hobby-related discussions.

· · · · ● · ● · · ·

# Self-Improvement and Skill Development

**Learning new skills and hobbies**

- Browse online courses, workshops, or local classes that pique your interest. They're like an all-you-can-learn buffet, so fill your plate with knowledge.

- Don't be afraid to try something completely new or outside your comfort zone. Remember, you once didn't know how to tie your shoes, and now you're a pro!

- Take your time and be patient with yourself. Rome wasn't built in a day, and neither will your new hobby expertise.

**Developing expertise in your chosen pursuits**

- Set specific, achievable goals to help you measure your progress and stay motivated.

- Seek out resources like books, online tutorials, and mentorship from experts to deepen your understanding and skill level.

- Practice, practice, practice! There's no substitute for hands-on experience, even if it means failing a few times (or a hundred) along the way.

**Overcoming the fear of failure**

- Embrace the idea of "failing forward." Each failure brings valuable lessons and experiences that help you grow.

- Share your journey with friends or online communities who can offer support, encouragement, and maybe even a few "I've been there!" stories.

- Remember, nobody's perfect. Even Beyoncé trips on stage sometimes, and she's still Queen Bey!

• • • ● • ● • • •

# Nature-Based Hobbies

## Hiking and Backpacking

"Forest bathing" (Shinrin-yoku) has been shown in studies to have a variety of health benefits, both physiological and psychological, including lowering blood pressure, enhancing autonomic and immune functions, relieving depression, and improving mental health.[1]

- Find trails that match your fitness level and desired solitude. There's no shame in being a "beginner" hiker or preferring quieter trails.

- Bring a friend or join a hiking group for added safety and companionship, but don't forget to soak in the peacefulness of nature.

- Invest in comfortable, reliable gear to make your outdoor adventures more enjoyable. Happy feet = happy hiker.

## Gardening

- Start small with a container garden or a few potted plants, and then work your way up to a full-blown backyard oasis.

- Choose plants that match your personality and lifestyle. Are you a low-maintenance cactus person or a high-maintenance rose aficionado?

- Connect with fellow gardeners online or in person for tips, tricks, and plant-swapping fun. Gardening friends are the best kind of enablers.

## Birdwatching

- Equip yourself with a good pair of binoculars, a field guide, and a sense of wonder for the avian world.

- Visit local parks, nature reserves, or even your own backyard to discover the fascinating lives of birds right under your nose (or, more accurately, above your head).

---

1. Furuyashiki A., Tabuchi K., Norikoshi K., Kobayashi T., And Oriyama S. - A comparative study of the physiological and psychological effects of forest bathing (Shinrin-yoku) on working age people with and without depressive tendencies (2019) https://www.ncbi.nlm.nih.gov/pmc/articles/PMC6589172/#:~:
text=Studies%20have%20found%20that%20%E2%80%9C
forest,depression%20and%20improving%20mental%20health.

- Join a local birdwatching group or participate in citizen science projects to share your sightings and contribute to our understanding of these feathered friends.

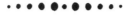

## Mindfulness-Based Hobbies

### Meditation and Yoga

- Explore different meditation and yoga styles to find the one that resonates with you. Remember, one person's "om" is another person's "ugh."

- Create a dedicated space in your home for your practice, even if it's just a small corner with a cushion or yoga mat.

- Be patient and kind to yourself as you cultivate your practice. Progress may be slow, but it's still progress.

### Coloring and Painting

- Choose a coloring book or painting subject that brings you joy, whether it's intricate mandalas, cute animals, or serene landscapes.

- Experiment with different mediums, like colored pencils, markers, or watercolors. You might discover a hidden talent or a new favorite pastime.

- Lose yourself in the creative process, allowing your mind to focus solely on the colors, shapes, and patterns before you.

### Journaling

- Decide on a journaling style that suits you, whether it's free writing, bullet journaling, or gratitude journaling. The world of journaling is your oyster!

- Find a notebook or journal that inspires you. Whether it's a simple composition book or a luxurious leather-bound tome, it should make you excited to write.

- Set aside time each day or week to reflect and write. Journaling can be a therapeutic way to process your thoughts and emotions in a safe space.

· · · · ●· ●· ● · ·

# Digital-Based Hobbies

### Online Gaming

- Discover your gaming preferences by exploring different genres, such as role-playing games (RPGs), strategy games, or puzzle games. There's something for everyone!

- Connect with other gamers through online forums or social media groups to share tips, strategies, and camaraderie.

- Remember to take breaks and practice good self-care. Gaming marathons can be fun, but don't forget to hydrate, stretch, and occasionally see the sun.

### Blogging and Writing

- Choose a topic or niche that you're passionate about, and start writing! Share your knowledge, experiences, or creative stories with the world.

- Develop your writing skills through online courses, workshops, or by simply writing consistently. Practice makes progress!

- Network with fellow bloggers and writers to learn from each other and form valuable connections in the digital world.

### Online Learning

- Explore the vast array of online courses, webinars, and tutorials available on nearly every subject imaginable. From coding to cooking, there's always something new to learn.

- Set realistic goals for your learning journey, and remember that it's okay to learn at your own pace. Slow and steady wins the race!

- Apply your newfound knowledge and skills to your life or career. You never know when that random course on ancient Egyptian history might come in handy (or at least make for interesting party conversation).

# CHAPTER SEVEN

---

# HOME SWEET HOME: CREATING A SANCTUARY FOR INTROVERTS AND HIGHLY SENSITIVE PEOPLE

---

T HERE'S NO PLACE LIKE home. For I/HSPs, home is not just where the heart is but also a place where they can recharge, rejuvenate, and be their true selves. Creating a sanctuary that promotes relaxation and harmony is essential for to thrive. In this chapter, we'll explore how to design and personalize your living space to make it the perfect oasis for you.

As an introvert or HSP, you may have a unique set of preferences when it comes to your living space. Factors such as lighting, noise levels, and color schemes can have a significant impact on your mood and overall well-being. We'll provide tips and guidance to help you transform your home into a sanctuary that reflects your personality and supports your needs.

· · · ● · ● · ● · ·

# Designing Your Space

Your home should be a reflection of who you are and what you love. For I/HSPs, designing a space that nurtures and inspires them is crucial. In this section, we'll discuss the importance of creating a personalized space that supports your introverted or highly sensitive nature. We'll also offer tips for decluttering and organizing, as well as incorporating elements of coziness and comfort to create a haven that feels like home.

### Designing a space that nurtures and inspires you

As an introvert or highly sensitive person, you may feel the effects of your environment more acutely than others. That's why it's so important to design a room around your specific likes, hobbies, and requirements. Here are some ideas for designing a space that nurtures and inspires you:

- **Choose a calming color palette:** Soft, muted colors are generally more soothing for I/HSPs. Consider using shades of blue, green, or gray for your walls, as they promote calmness and relaxation.

- **Incorporate natural elements:** Bringing nature into your home can have a positive effect on your mental health. Include plants, natural materials such as wood and stone, and artwork featuring natural landscapes to create a serene atmosphere.

- **Create designated quiet spaces:** Designate specific areas in your home for quiet activities, such as reading, meditation, or journaling. This will provide you with a place to retreat and recharge when you need some alone time.

### Tips for decluttering and organizing

A clutter-free environment can have a significant impact on your mental well-being, especially for I/HSPs, who are often more affected by their surroundings. Here are some tips for decluttering and organizing your space:

1. **Start small:** Tackle one area at a time, such as a closet, drawer, or shelf. Breaking the process down into smaller tasks can make decluttering feel less overwhelming.

2. **Use the KonMari Method:** Marie Kondo's popular organizing method[1] involves keeping items that "spark joy" and discarding those that do not. This can be a helpful approach for I/HSPs, as it encourages you to surround yourself with things that bring you happiness and have meaning.

3. **Implement storage solutions:** Use storage solutions such as shelves, baskets, and bins to keep your belongings organized and easily accessible.

· · · ● ●· ● ● · ·

## Incorporating elements of coziness and comfort

A cozy and comfortable home can be incredibly soothing for I/HSPs. Here are some suggestions for creating a warm and inviting atmosphere:

- **Soft lighting:** Harsh lighting can be overstimulating for I/HSPs. Opt for lamps with warm-toned bulbs and consider adding dimmer switches to control the intensity of your lighting. You can also use candles or string lights to create a cozy ambiance.

- **Comfortable seating:** Invest in comfortable furniture that supports relaxation, such as a plush sofa, a reading chair, or a window seat. Adding plenty of pillows and throws can also contribute to a cozy atmosphere.

- **Incorporate textures:** Layering different textures, such as soft rugs, blankets, and curtains, can create a sense of warmth and comfort in your space.

- **Personalize your space:** Display meaningful items, such as family photos, artwork, or mementos from your travels, to make your home feel more personal and inviting.

- **Create a sensory haven:** Create a relaxing atmosphere that engages all of your

---

1. Kondo, M. (2014). The life-changing magic of tidying up: The Japanese art of decluttering and organizing. Ten Speed Press.

senses by using essential oil diffusers, scented candles, and relaxing music or sounds of nature.

Now that you know how to create a safe and uplifting environment, you can focus on decluttering and organizing your home to better accommodate your introverted or highly sensitive personality. In the following section, we'll go over some practical tips and strategies for creating a clutter-free and organized living space that promotes relaxation and well-being.

· · · ●·●·● · · ·

## Creating a Calming Atmosphere

Introverts and people with high levels of sensitivity need a quiet place to recharge and relax at home, so it's important to make your home a calm place. In this section, we'll talk about how to choose colors, lighting, and smells that are soothing to your senses, how to make a quiet and peaceful space, and how to add plants and other natural elements to your home. Using these suggestions as a starting point, you can design a private space that perfectly suits your tastes and preferences.

### Selecting colors, lighting, and scents that soothe your senses

Your home's color scheme, lighting scheme, and aroma all have an effect on your state of mind and general well-being. Here are some guidelines for picking out furnishings that will help create a relaxing ambiance:

- **Colors:** Choose soothing tones such as light blues, greens, and grays. These colors have been shown to induce feelings of calm and peace. If you're an introvert or highly sensitive person, it's best to stay away from extremely bright or bold colors.

- **Lighting:** Use dimmable, warm lighting to set a relaxing mood. Lighting should be soft, so use lamps instead of overhead lights if possible. When you need to relax and unwind without being disturbed by bright sunlight, closing the blinds or curtains can help.

- **Scents:** Aromatherapy is a great way to set the mood for relaxation. Oils extracted from plants, such as lavender, chamomile, and bergamot, have long been used for their sedative and relaxing effects. Spread these calming aromas throughout your home with a diffuser or some scented candles.

## Creating a quiet and peaceful environment

Introverts and people with high levels of sensitivity require a peaceful setting in which to recharge and stay healthy. Here are some methods for making a calm environment:

- **Soundproofing:** Soundproof your home by installing acoustic panels or foam on walls, adding sound-absorbing rugs and curtains, and weatherstripping your doors and windows.

- **Quiet appliances:** The noise level in your home can be reduced by selecting appliances with a low decibel rating. Try to find appliances like washing machines, dryers, and air cleaners that boast a "quiet" or "silent" setting.

- **Designated quiet zones:** Make sure you have a place to go to get some peace and quiet at home. This could be a quiet corner for reading or contemplation, or even a whole room set aside for such pursuits.

## Incorporating plants and natural elements

There are many ways in which the addition of plants and other natural elements to your home can improve your emotional and physical well-being. Here are some tips for integrating nature into your home:

- **Indoor plants:** Having plants around the house has many benefits, including better air quality, less stress, and a better mood. If you're just starting out, select low-maintenance plants like snake plants, pothos, or ZZ plants.

- **Natural materials:** Connect with the outdoors by furnishing and decorating with natural materials like wood, stone, and wicker. This can help create a calming and grounding atmosphere.

- **Nature-inspired artwork:** Put up paintings or photographs of serene natural settings like forests, mountains, or beaches to help you relax at home.

- **Water features:** If you're looking to add some tranquility to your space, one option is to set up a small water feature, such as a tabletop fountain or an aquarium.

With these methods in place, you can make your house a sanctuary for your introverted or highly sensitive self. Next, we'll talk about how to strike the right balance between public and private areas in your home to suit your lifestyle.

· · · ● · ● · ● · ·

## Balancing Social and Private Spaces

Even though I/HSPs need their alone time, it's important to have a mix of social and private areas in your house. This balance allows you to comfortably host gatherings and socialize with friends and family while also providing dedicated areas for solitude and reflection. This section will go over how to design areas for hosting and socializing, how to create a dedicated space for solitude and reflection, and how to maintain privacy in shared living situations.

### Designing areas for hosting and socializing

Social gathering places are important for everyone, and that includes introverts and people with high levels of sensitivity. Some ideas for making your home more inviting in social settings:

- **Dedicated gathering spaces:** Set aside specific rooms or outdoor spaces for hosting guests. Add some coziness to these areas by furnishing them with plenty of seating, low lighting, and warm accents.

- **Flexible furniture arrangements:** Pick out flexible seating that can easily be moved around to accommodate a wide range of group sizes and uses. Expandable tables, modular seating, and folding chairs are all great choices.

- **Consider traffic flow:** Position the furniture so that it won't get in the way of anyone while they're talking. Make sure there's plenty of room for people to move around and set up conversation areas with seating facing inwards.

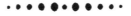

## Creating a dedicated space for solitude and reflection

A dedicated space for solitude and reflection is crucial for I/HSPs. Here are some ideas for creating a private retreat in your home:

- **Choose a quiet location:** Choose a secluded spot at home, whether it's an unused bedroom, a section of the living room, or even a walk-in closet, and devote it to your need for personal time and reflection.

- **Incorporate calming elements:** Create a relaxing environment in your personal space by filling it with warm, comforting features.

- **Personalize your space:** Put together a cozy space by surrounding yourself with things that make you happy, such as artwork, mementos, and books.

### Tips for maintaining privacy in shared living situations

For introverts and people with high levels of sensitivity, maintaining privacy can be especially difficult in shared living situations. Some suggestions for maintaining personal space in a shared dwelling:

- **Set boundaries:** Make your privacy needs known to your roommates so that everyone knows where they stand. Share your need for peace and quiet and work together to establish quiet "quiet hours" or spaces in your home.

- **Use room dividers:** Folding screens and bookshelves are just two examples of room dividers that can be used to create acoustic and visual privacy in otherwise open areas.

- **Invest in noise-canceling headphones:** Living with others can be challenging for I/HSPs, but noise-canceling headphones or even regular earplugs can be a lifesaver. When you need some peace and quiet, they can help you achieve that by creating a sense of privacy and blocking out noise.

By arranging your home with a healthy mix of public and private areas, you can create a haven that supports your introverted or highly sensitive personality while still facilitating meaningful interactions with friends and family. With these tips and strategies, you can transform your living space into a haven that supports your unique needs and preferences.

# CHAPTER EIGHT

## TRAVELING AND EXPLORING THE WORLD AS AN INTROVERT AND HSP

For I/HSPs, traveling the world and experiencing new cultures can be an enriching but also taxing endeavor. It's important to strike a balance between exploring new places and taking care of yourself when traveling.

In this chapter, we will discuss how to prepare for a trip, handle social situations while away, and open yourself up to new experiences if you are an introvert or highly sensitive person. With a little planning and self-awareness, you can create a travel experience that nourishes your soul, expands your horizons, and leaves you feeling refreshed and inspired.

## Planning Your Trip

Planning ahead is essential for I/HSPs to have a relaxing and enjoyable vacation. You can make your trip more enjoyable by planning ahead for things like lodging, transportation, and the kinds of things you need to bring with you.

**Tips for planning a trip that suits your needs**

1. **Define your travel goals:** Think about what you hope to get out of your vacation before you start making plans. Do you want to kick back and relax, or experience the local culture? Would you like to travel alone, with someone else,

or with a group? Having a clear idea of your preferences before booking a trip will help you pick the perfect location, activities, and lodging.

2. **Choose the right destination:** Although visits to busy cities and other popular tourist destinations often provide memorable experiences, they may not be optimal for introverts and those with heightened sensitivity. Think about places that offer a more laid-back vibe, such as those rich in natural beauty. This could be a sleepy seaside community, a quaint mountain hamlet, or a tranquil retreat.

3. **Timing is key:** It's best to plan trips during the shoulder or off-peak seasons to avoid the worst of the crowds and the most intense levels of activity. You'll find fewer people traveling at the same time, and you might even save money on lodging and transportation.

4. **Research accommodations carefully:** Look for a place to stay that offers peace and quiet and some privacy. Look for hotels, guesthouses, or vacation rentals that cater to I/HSPs, or simply seek out accommodations with private balconies, gardens, or quiet common areas. Read reviews to learn about the noise levels and overall atmosphere of the place.

5. **Create a flexible itinerary:** While preparation is key, so is the ability to adapt to change. Include some downtime in your schedule to refresh and refocus. It's important to give yourself time to relax, whether that's in your hotel room, a nearby park, or a quaint café.

· · · · ● · ● · · ·

## Researching destinations and accommodations

1. **Utilize online resources:** Websites like TripAdvisor, Lonely Planet, and Fodor's can provide invaluable information about potential destinations and accommodations. Read reviews from other travelers, particularly those who identify as introverts or HSPs, to get a sense of what to expect.

2. **Reach out to local experts:** Connecting with locals or experts in the area

can help you uncover hidden gems and quiet spots that may not be listed in guidebooks. This can be done through social media, travel forums, or even reaching out to local tourism offices.

3. **Consider alternative accommodations:** If traditional hotels or hostels don't seem appealing, look into alternative options like vacation rentals (e.g., Airbnb), boutique hotels, or even monasteries and retreat centers that offer guest accommodations. These options can provide a more personalized, quiet, and peaceful experience.

• • • ● • ● • • •

## Packing essentials for I/HSPs

1. **Noise-canceling headphones:** Noise-canceling headphones can be used to block out unwanted noise on flights, in airports, or at crowded attractions. They can give you a much-needed break from overstimulation and help you stay calm.

2. **Comfort items:** Bring a few items from home that bring you comfort, such as a soft scarf, your favorite tea, or a familiar book. These items can help you feel more at ease in unfamiliar surroundings.

3. **Travel journal:** A journal can be an excellent tool for processing your experiences, reflecting on your day, and expressing your thoughts and feelings. It can also serve as a memento of your travels.

4. **Sensory aids:** If you're highly sensitive to certain stimuli, pack items that can help you manage sensory overload, such as earplugs, an eye mask, or calming essential oils.

5. **Portable charger:** A portable charger ensures your devices are always charged, so you can access maps, translation apps, and other helpful resources when you need them.

6. **Entertainment:** Load your phone, tablet, or e-reader with books, podcasts, or

movies to keep you entertained during downtime or when you need a break from socializing.

With a solid plan, the right destination, and a suitcase filled with essential items, you'll be well-prepared for a fulfilling and enjoyable trip that caters to your introverted or highly sensitive nature. In the following section, we'll go over how to navigate social interactions while traveling so you can connect with others and make the most of your trip.

· · · · ● · ● · · ·

## Navigating Social Interactions While Traveling

When you travel, you'll likely encounter new people, cultures, and social situations that you'll need to learn how to handle. For I/HSPs, these social interactions can be both rewarding and challenging. In this section, I'll provide tips for overcoming language barriers, making connections with fellow travelers and locals, and balancing social time with alone time.

### Overcoming language barriers and cultural differences

1. **Learn key phrases:** Before you travel, familiarize yourself with basic phrases in the local language, such as greetings, "please" and "thank you," and essential questions. Even a small effort to speak the local language can go a long way in making connections and showing respect for the local culture.

2. **Use translation apps:** Download a translation app like Google Translate on your phone to help you communicate more effectively. This can be particularly useful when navigating public transportation, ordering food, or asking for directions.

3. **Do your research:** Learn about the local customs, etiquette, and social norms before your trip. This will help you feel more at ease in social situations and minimize the risk of unintentionally offending someone.

4. **Be open and adaptable:** Embrace the differences in language and culture as an

opportunity to learn and grow. Approach new experiences with curiosity and an open mind, and be willing to adapt to unfamiliar situations.

$$\bullet \; \bullet \; \bullet \; \bullet \; \bullet \; \bullet \; \bullet \; \bullet \; \bullet \; \bullet$$

## Making connections with fellow travelers and locals

1. **Select social activities based on your interests:** Engage in activities that align with your passions and interests, such as cooking classes, art workshops, or guided nature walks. These activities will naturally attract like-minded people, making it easier to strike up conversations and form connections.

2. **Utilize online platforms**: Social media and travel forums can be excellent tools for connecting with fellow travelers or locals. You can join groups dedicated to your destination or interest, or use apps like Meetup to find events and gatherings.

3. **Stay in smaller, intimate accommodations:** Choosing smaller hotels, guesthouses, or bed and breakfasts can provide more opportunities for meaningful interactions with fellow guests and hosts.

4. **Stay present:** When engaging in conversations, focus on truly listening and empathizing with the other person. This can help create deeper connections and make the conversation more enjoyable for both parties.

$$\bullet \; \bullet \; \bullet \; \bullet \; \bullet \; \bullet \; \bullet \; \bullet \; \bullet \; \bullet$$

## Balancing social time with alone time

1. **Schedule downtime:** As an introvert or HSP, it's essential to prioritize downtime and self-care. Schedule regular breaks in your itinerary to recharge and reflect on your experiences.

2. **Set boundaries:** Be honest with yourself and others about your need for alone time. It's okay to decline invitations or let your travel companions know when you need some space.

3. **Seek out quiet spaces:** During your travels, find places where you can escape the noise and crowds, such as parks, gardens, or quiet cafés. These spaces can provide a much-needed sanctuary when you're feeling overwhelmed.

4. **Embrace solo activities:** Make time for activities that you enjoy doing alone, such as reading, journaling, or exploring a museum at your own pace. These activities can help you recharge and maintain a sense of balance during your trip.

These guidelines will help you handle social situations with ease and grace while traveling, allowing you to make new friends and unforgettable memories. Next, we'll look at some strategies for taking risks and trying new things, even if you're an introvert or highly sensitive person.

· · · · ● · ● · · ·

# Embracing Adventure and New Experiences

When you travel, you get to see the world, experience new things, and develop as a person. Adventure and new experiences can be both thrilling and terrifying for an introvert or HSP. Here we'll go over some ways to challenge yourself, record your experiences, and come back from a trip feeling more like your true self.

**Stepping out of your comfort zone**

1. **Set realistic goals:** Make a list of things you'd like to do or see while on your trip, and make sure they're within your reach. Something as simple as eating at a new restaurant, going on a guided tour, or dancing the local way qualifies. Having defined objectives can serve as a source of inspiration and drive.

2. **Start small:** Be patient with yourself and ease into new situations by taking on less daunting tasks first. Your bravery and flexibility will grow as you take on

ever-greater challenges.

3. **Find a travel buddy:** Talk to the people you're traveling with about what you hope to get out of the trip, and push each other to try new things. If you're traveling solo, having someone who will encourage you can be a huge confidence boost.

4. **Embrace vulnerability:** Recognize that it is normal to experience anxiety when confronted with something unfamiliar. It is okay to feel these emotions as a natural part of the development process. Remember that it is a great chance for you to learn and grow.

· · · ● · ● · · ·

## Capturing memories and reflecting on your journey

1. **Document your experiences:** Keep a travel journal or blog to record your thoughts, feelings, and experiences. This can help you process and reflect on your journey, as well as create a lasting keepsake.

2. **Take photos**: Capture the beauty and wonder of your travels through photography. Experiment with different angles, lighting, and subjects to create a visual narrative of your trip.

3. **Collect mementos:** Save small tokens from your travels, such as postcards, ticket stubs, or local handicrafts. These items can serve as tangible reminders of your experiences and personal growth.

4. **Share your story:** Share your travel experiences with friends, family, or online communities. This can help you reflect on your journey, connect with others who share your interests, and inspire others to embark on their own adventures.

· · · ● · ● · ● · ·

## Returning home with a renewed sense of self

1. **Integrate your experiences:** As you return home, consider how your travels have impacted your perspective, values, and priorities. Look for ways to incorporate the lessons and experiences from your trip into your daily life.

2. **Stay connected:** Maintain relationships with the people you've met during your travels, whether they're fellow travelers or locals. These connections can enrich your life and provide ongoing support and inspiration.

3. **Continue exploring:** Embrace the spirit of adventure and curiosity in your everyday life by seeking out new experiences and challenges at home. This can help you maintain the personal growth and sense of renewal you experienced while traveling.

4. **Plan your next adventure:** Reflect on the aspects of your trip that you enjoyed the most, and use this insight to plan future travels that align with your interests and needs as an introvert or HSP.

Taking risks and trying new things is a great way to develop as a person and make memories that will last a lifetime. For those who are more introverted or highly sensitive, traveling can be a life-changing experience that allows them to branch out of their comfort zones, build meaningful relationships, and return home with a refreshed perspective on who they are.

# CHAPTER NINE

## OVERCOMING OBSTACLES AND EMBRACING CHANGE

L IFE IS FILLED WITH challenges and changes, and as an introvert or HSP, these situations can sometimes feel overwhelming or downright terrifying. But don't worry! You are capable of overcoming challenges and adjusting to new situations because of your strength and resilience. In this section, I'll teach you how to solve problems, adjust to new circumstances, and reflect on your progress. Developing these skills will make you more resilient to life's ups and downs and more likely to achieve your goals.

## Developing Problem-Solving Skills

Whether it's a setback in your career, a rift with a loved one, or an unexpected financial obstacle, difficulties will arise. I/HSPs might internalize these issues, leading to stress and anxiety. You can, however, overcome challenges by cultivating effective problem-solving skills.

### Analyzing Challenges and Brainstorming Solutions

The first thing to do when trying to solve a problem is to break it down and look at its parts. This process can help you figure out what's really going on and come up with possible solutions. As an introvert or HSP, you have a natural ability to think deeply and reflectively, which can be an asset in this phase of problem-solving.

**Lena's story:**

Lena, an introverted person with high levels of sensitivity, was dealing with a situation at work that was incredibly stressful for her. Her team had just been given a new project with extremely short deadlines, and the pressure to produce high-quality work as quickly as possible was getting to her. Lena decided to take a methodical approach to solving the problem.

**Define the problem:** Lena started by describing the problem she was having. She realized that the pressure was building up because of the short deadlines, the weight of the expectations, and her desire for uninterrupted work time.

**Gather information:** Lena gathered data and context to help her comprehend the issue at hand. She looked over the project specifications, questioned her colleagues about their own similar experiences, and investigated methods of time and task management.

Lena relied on her analytical and introspective tendencies to come up with a list of potential solutions. She gave some thought to strategies such as subdividing the work into more manageable chunks, enlisting help from others, and blocking off time each day to focus on the project at hand.

**Evaluate the options:** Then, Lena weighed the benefits and drawbacks of each option, considering things like how much time and money it would take to implement. While asking for more resources might be impossible under the current circumstances, she saw that breaking the project into smaller tasks and setting aside quiet hours were the most feasible options.

**Choose a course of action:** Based on her evaluation, Lena decided to break the project into smaller tasks and establish quiet hours during the day. In addition to managing tight deadlines and high expectations more efficiently and effectively, she felt confident that these solutions would help her.

Following this method, Lena was able to handle the stressful work environment and meet her project deadlines without sacrificing her well-being as an introvert.

• • • ● • ● • • •

## Seeking Help and Advice When Needed

Although I/HSPs tend to rely on their own resources, they still need to know when to ask for assistance. Seeking help is not a sign of weakness, and it can help you see things from angles you hadn't considered before. Get in touch with people you know who may have dealt with a similar situation in the past, or think about consulting a trained expert like a therapist or career coach. Don't be embarrassed to reach out for assistance; doing so demonstrates strength and maturity.

### Learning from Mistakes and Setbacks

Nobody's perfect, and we all have to deal with failures and mistakes. Learning from adversity and using it to improve oneself is essential for success. If you're an introvert or highly sensitive person, you probably learn a lot from thinking deeply about the world and how it works. Consider what went wrong and how things could be improved for the future. Doing so will help you become more resilient and resourceful in the face of adversity in the future.

• • • ● • ● • • •

## Adapting to New Situations

There are many transitions in life, including beginning a new job, relocating to a new city, or the end of a relationship. As an introvert or HSP, adapting to new situations can be challenging, as you may feel overwhelmed by the unknown and crave the comfort of familiarity. But you can learn to welcome the unexpected and tap into the potential for self-improvement that comes with navigating life's changes by developing resilience and coping strategies.

### Navigating Major Life Changes and Transitions

Whether you're facing a significant life change or simply adjusting to a new routine, it's essential to approach the situation with a positive mindset and a willingness to adapt.

**Mason's story:**

For the shy Mason, a great job opportunity had just opened up in a different city across the country. He was thrilled by the prospect of this new venture, but he was also worried about the difficulties of settling into a completely new lifestyle and set of friends. Mason made the decision to follow some helpful guidelines to assist him in making this significant life change.

**Acknowledge your feelings:** As Mason began to prepare for his move, he experienced a mix of emotions, from excitement about the new job to anxiety about leaving his familiar surroundings. Recognizing that it was normal to experience such emotions during a time of profound personal transition, he gave himself permission to accept and embrace them.

**Set realistic expectations:** Mason knew that adjusting to his new life would take time and that it was normal to experience some discomfort or uncertainty along the way. He prepared himself for the fact that it would take some time before he felt at home in his new city.

**Break the change down into manageable steps:** Mason took the transition one step at a time to make it more manageable for himself and his family. He set small, achievable goals, such as finding a new apartment, registering for a local gym, and exploring his new neighborhood. These goals gradually helped him adjust to his new situation.

**Stay flexible:** Throughout the process, Mason remained open to the idea that his plans and expectations might need to change as he adapted to his new circumstances. For instance, after doing some investigating, he realized that a different area was better suited to his needs and preferences than the one he had originally planned to move to. Because of his adaptability, he was able to handle unexpected situations with relative ease.

Mason was able to make the big move and adjust to his new city with the help of these tips. He settled into his new routine and began to enjoy himself, finally able to take advantage of all the wonderful possibilities his new job and lifestyle presented.

· · · ● · ● · · ·

## Building Resilience and Coping Skills

Like a rollercoaster, life has its ups and downs, turns and twists, and even some unexpected detours. Problems and failures are a part of life no matter who you are or where you come from. These challenges can be especially trying for I/HSPs, who typically have heightened emotional sensitivity and a predisposition toward introspection. So, building resilience and practicing coping skills are important if you want to handle life's challenges with poise and strength.

Resilience is the ability to get back up after a setback, adapt to change, and keep your balance when you're under a lot of stress. It is a trait that allows people to keep going even when things get hard. Some people may be more resilient by nature, but it's important to remember that this is not a trait that everyone has. Instead, it's a skill that can be learned and improved over time.

On the other hand, coping skills are the specific strategies and techniques that people use to deal with stress, get through hard times, and keep their emotional health in check. These skills can range from simple ways to relax to more complicated ways to solve problems. Like resilience, coping skills can be learned and improved with practice and thought.

For I/HSPs, building resilience and improving coping skills can be especially important because they often experience the world in a more intense and profound way. By building a strong foundation of resilience and honing their coping skills, I/HSPs can better handle the challenges that life throws at them, allowing them to thrive in the face of adversity and embrace personal growth.

**Sophie's story:**

Sophie, an HSP, had to deal with a number of problems in her personal and professional life. She knew that to get past these problems, she needed to get stronger and get better at dealing with things. She decided to do this by using a set of strategies that were made for I/HSPs.

**Fostering a strong support network:** Sophie realized that having a solid support network was crucial for her well-being. She began by reaching out to her friends, family, and other loved ones, opening up about the challenges she was facing. During her hard times, she found that they were more than willing to cheer her up, give her advice, and just listen to her. Sophie also joined a local support group for I/HSPs so she could meet other people like her and talk about her experiences.

**Practicing self-care:** Sophie understood that prioritizing her physical, emotional, and mental well-being was essential for building resilience. She made a plan for taking care of herself that included regular exercise, doing things she enjoyed, and practicing ways to relax like meditation and deep breathing. This routine helped her stay healthy even though things were hard.

**Maintaining a positive mindset:** Sophie made a conscious effort to focus on her strengths and accomplishments rather than dwelling on the negative aspects of her situation. She reminded herself that she had dealt with problems in the past and changed her attitude about life. This way of thinking gave her the confidence and strength she needed to deal with her problems.

**Learning from past experiences:** To further develop her resilience, Sophie reflected on her previous experiences with change and adversity. She thought about what helped her adjust in the past and what she could do differently this time. She realized, for example, that she had often tried to handle everything on her own in the past, which only made her more stressed. This time, she decided to ask for help and support when she needed it. This made her stronger and better able to deal with the problems she was facing.

Sophie improved her ability to cope as an HSP by developing her resilience through the use of these methods. She overcame challenges and adjusted to life changes with ease and confidence thanks to her strong support system, dedication to self-care, optimistic outlook, and ability to learn from past experiences.

• • • • ● • ● • • •

# Embracing the Unknown and the Power of Personal Growth

Change can help you grow as a person by pushing you to learn new skills, broaden your horizons, and find strengths you didn't know you had. Embrace the unknown by:

1. **Viewing change as an opportunity:** Try to see the potential for growth and self-improvement in every new situation, rather than focusing solely on the challenges or discomfort.

2. **Being open to new experiences:** Push yourself to try new things and step outside of your comfort zone, even if it feels scary or intimidating at first.

3. **Celebrating your progress:** Acknowledge and celebrate your achievements, no matter how small, as you navigate the transition. This can help boost your confidence and reinforce your ability to adapt.

. . . ● . ● . . .

# Celebrating Your Journey

Throughout your journey of adulting as an introvert or HSP, it's important to take the time to recognize and celebrate your achievements, both big and small. Recognizing your growth and progress is a great way to boost your self-esteem and keep a positive attitude as you face more challenges in life. In this section, we'll talk about how important it is to celebrate your journey, be kind to yourself, and grow self-love.

### Recognizing and Celebrating Your Achievements

Sometimes, we can get so caught up in the problems and challenges that we forget to celebrate the things we've done well. As an introvert or HSP, it's important to take the time to celebrate your successes. Here are some ways to do that:

1. **Keep a success journal:** Regularly jot down your accomplishments, both big and small. This will serve as a visual reminder of your progress and can be a source of motivation during difficult times.

2. **Reward yourself:** Treat yourself to something special when you reach a milestone or accomplish a goal. This can be anything from a favorite dessert to a weekend getaway.

3. **Share your achievements with others:** Don't hesitate to share your successes with friends and family. They can offer encouragement and support, helping to reinforce your accomplishments.

· · · **·** · **·** · · ·

## Acknowledging Your Growth and Progress

Personal growth is a journey that never ends, and it's important to keep track of the steps you've taken along the way. Think about how you've changed, the skills you've gained, and the problems you've solved. Recognizing your progress can help you keep a positive attitude and motivate you to keep trying to get better.

**Embracing Self-Compassion and Self-Love**

As an introvert or HSP, you may be particularly prone to self-criticism and negative self-talk. However, it's essential to embrace self-compassion and self-love as you navigate the journey of adulting. Here are some strategies for cultivating self-compassion and self-love:

1. **Practice self-compassion:** Treat yourself with the same kindness and understanding that you would offer a friend in a similar situation. Recognize that everyone makes mistakes and faces challenges, and it's okay to be imperfect.

2. **Challenge negative self-talk:** When you notice self-critical thoughts creeping in, challenge them by asking yourself whether they're accurate, helpful, or fair. Replace these negative thoughts with more compassionate, supportive statements.

3. **Make time for self-care:** Regularly engage in activities that bring you joy, relaxation, and a sense of accomplishment. Prioritizing self-care is a crucial

component of self-love and can contribute to overall well-being.

In this section, we've explored the importance of celebrating your journey as an introvert or HSP, including recognizing and celebrating your achievements, acknowledging your growth and progress, and embracing self-compassion and self-love. By implementing these strategies, you can cultivate a more positive, compassionate attitude towards yourself, leading to greater confidence and resilience as you continue your journey of adulting.

# CHAPTER TEN

## BUILDING A SUPPORTIVE COMMUNITY

I N TODAY'S FAST-PACED AND often chaotic world, it's more important than ever to build a community of people who care about each other. This can be especially hard for I/HSPs, who may need more time alone and attention to their surroundings than their more outgoing peers. But it's important to have a strong network of like-minded people to help you deal with life's challenges, grow as a person, and find happiness and well-being.

A community that helps each other out gives people a safe place to talk about their lives, share ideas, and cheer each other on. It's a place where I/HSPs can feel understood, accepted, and valued for their unique qualities. Also, a supportive community can help people deal with the stresses of daily life and improve their emotional health.

In addition to emotional support, a strong community gives people chances to grow and develop. I/HSPs can learn more, improve their skills, and gain new perspectives by connecting with people who have similar interests, values, and experiences. This can be especially helpful for people who have trouble finding their place in a world that often values outgoing qualities and actions.

Creating a supportive community also helps people feel like they belong and are connected, which is important for happiness and mental health as a whole. For I/HSPs, finding a group of like-minded individuals can provide a much-needed sense of belonging, which can positively impact their emotional well-being and overall life satisfaction.

A supportive community can also offer help and resources when they are needed. Whether it's a helping hand during a difficult time or valuable advice on navigating life's challenges, the support of a caring community can make a significant difference in the lives of I/HSPs. By collaborating with others and contributing to the well-being of the community, they can also experience a sense of purpose and fulfillment.

· · · ● · ● · ● · ·

## Finding Like-Minded Individuals

### Joining clubs and organizations for I/HSPs

One way to find a group of people who will support you is to join clubs and organizations that are made for I/HSPs. These groups understand and meet the individual needs of their members, making it easy for them to make friends and grow as people.

### Meet Sarah.

Sarah is a highly sensitive introvert who has always found it difficult to connect with people. She realized that finding like-minded individuals would make her journey through adulting more enjoyable. She decided to join a local club for I/HSPs. She looked for support groups online and found a lot of them all over the world. She was nervous at first about going to the meetings, but she soon realized that the atmosphere was calm, quiet, and friendly. She found that the group members understood and respected each other's boundaries, which let her open up and talk about her experiences without feeling too much.

### Utilizing online platforms and social media to connect with others

Online platforms and social media are great ways to find people with similar interests. There are a lot of groups, forums, and communities for introverts and people with high sensitivity. These online spaces provide opportunities to share experiences, exchange ideas, and form friendships without the pressure of face-to-face interactions.

### Attending meetups and events tailored to your interests

Participating in meetups and events centered around your interests is another way to find a supportive community. Look for gatherings specifically designed for I/HSPs, where the atmosphere is calm and welcoming. Engaging with others who share your passions will make it easier to form meaningful connections.

Anna is an HSP who loves reading and discussing books. She discovered a local book club through the Meetup app, which focused on creating a peaceful and welcoming environment for I/HSPs. The group would meet at a cozy, quiet café once a month to discuss a selected book. Anna found that the relaxed atmosphere and shared love for literature helped her form deep connections with the other members.

· · · ● · ● · ● · · ·

## Fostering Meaningful Connections

### Cultivating deep friendships and relationships

Individuals who prefer quieter and more introspective experiences should prioritize meaningful friendships and connections over building a large social network. Focusing on quality rather than quantity, it becomes important to spend time and energy building relationships with people who truly understand and value your unique qualities.

David, an introvert with a passion for photography, met his now-best-friend, Emma, at a photography workshop. They connected over their shared love for nature photography, and their friendship blossomed. They made a pact to schedule monthly photo walks to different parks and nature reserves. Through these shared experiences, David and Emma have cultivated a deep, meaningful friendship, which has provided them both with a strong support system.

### Strengthening bonds through shared experiences

Shared experiences can help strengthen the bonds between I/HSPs. Participating in activities, hobbies, or projects together will provide opportunities to connect on a deeper level and create lasting memories.

Susan and Tom, a highly sensitive couple, have always valued their emotional connection. To strengthen their bond, they decided to take up a hobby together—pottery. They enrolled in a pottery class at a local community center, and they found that working side-by-side on a creative project brought them even closer. As they shared their triumphs and struggles, they were able to support and encourage each other, fostering a deeper understanding and appreciation for one another.

### Nurturing a sense of belonging and support

A sense of belonging and support is crucial as you navigate through life. Make an effort to maintain regular contact with your close friends and family, and don't hesitate to reach out for help or encouragement when needed.

· · · · ● · ● · · ·

## Collaborating and Supporting Others

### Volunteering and giving back to your community

Volunteering is a fantastic way to give back to your community while also building a supportive network. Look for opportunities to contribute your skills and talents to causes that align with your values and interests. In doing so, you'll not only make a difference but also connect with others who share your passions.

### Lending a listening ear or offering advice

As an I/HSP, your empathetic nature and keen listening skills can be invaluable to others. Offer a listening ear or advice to friends, family, or even strangers in need. This act of kindness can deepen connections and foster a sense of community.

### Participating in group projects and activities

While group projects and activities may seem daunting to people like us, they can also be an opportunity for collaboration and support. Look for group endeavors that align with your interests and values, and approach them with an open mind. By working together with others, you'll not only achieve a common goal but also build a supportive community in the process.

# CHAPTER ELEVEN

## ASSERTIVENESS AND BOUNDARIES

I N A SOCIETY THAT often rewards extroversion and assertive behavior, I/HSPs may struggle to assert themselves and establish healthy boundaries in various aspects of their lives.

For people like us, the prospect of asserting ourselves or setting boundaries can be daunting. It may evoke feelings of guilt, discomfort, or even anxiety. We might worry about the reactions of others, the potential for conflict, or the perceived selfishness of putting our needs first. However, assertiveness and healthy boundaries are essential for maintaining our emotional well-being, protecting our energy, and fostering meaningful connections with others.

In this chapter, we'll talk about how important it is to learn how to be assertive and set healthy boundaries. We'll talk about practical ways to say what you need and want, get over your fear of confrontation, and set and stick to your own limits. Also, we'll talk about how to handle conflict and difficult situations. We'll talk about how to approach disagreements with empathy and understanding, how to solve conflicts well, and how to take criticism and feedback with grace.

As you read this chapter, keep in mind that being assertive is not the same as being mean or selfish. It's about taking care of your own feelings and needs while also being kind to other people. By learning to be assertive and setting healthy boundaries, you give yourself the tools you need to handle the complicated parts of being an adult. This gives you more self-confidence, self-respect, and well-being.

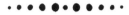

## Developing Assertiveness Skills

### Recognizing the importance of assertiveness

As an introvert or HSP, it's crucial to develop assertiveness skills. Being assertive allows you to:

- Stand up for your rights and beliefs without infringing on others'

- Communicate your needs and desires effectively

- Build healthy, respectful relationships

- Enhance self-esteem and self-confidence

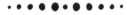

## Techniques for expressing your needs and desires

1. **Use "I" statements:** Focus on expressing your feelings and needs without blaming or accusing others. For example, instead of saying "You never listen to me," say "I feel ignored when you don't pay attention to what I'm saying."

2. **Practice active listening:** Show genuine interest in the other person's perspective by making eye contact, nodding, and asking open-ended questions. This demonstrates respect and encourages open communication.

3. **Be clear and concise:** Clearly articulate your needs, feelings, and opinions, without being overly verbose. This helps others understand your perspective

and increases the chances of your message being heard.

4. **Maintain a calm and confident tone:** Speak in a steady, calm tone and maintain a confident posture. This conveys self-assurance and helps keep the conversation on track.

5. **Use assertive body language:** Maintain eye contact, stand or sit straight, and use open gestures to convey confidence and self-assurance.

· · • • •• • •• • • ·

## Overcoming the fear of confrontation

Confrontation can be particularly challenging for us. However, it's important to remember that assertiveness is not aggression. Here are some tips to help you overcome the fear of confrontation:

- Reframe confrontation as an opportunity for growth and understanding

- Visualize a successful outcome before engaging in a difficult conversation

- Practice deep breathing or other relaxation techniques to manage anxiety

- Role-play confrontational scenarios with a trusted friend or therapist

Emily, a 27-year-old introverted and highly sensitive woman, had always dreaded confrontations. As a project manager at a marketing company, she often avoided hard conversations with her coworkers, even when they were important for the success of their projects. She felt frustrated and overwhelmed because she was afraid of confrontation. She knew that her inability to talk about problems was hurting her professional relationships and the quality of her work.

One day, a big project was at risk because team members didn't talk to each other well. Emily knew she had to face the problem head-on to stop any more delays, but she didn't because she was afraid of a fight. She decided to seek advice from her friend Sarah, who was known for her ability to handle confrontations with grace and assertiveness.

Sarah listened to Emily's worries with understanding and gave her some tips on how to get over being afraid of confrontation. She told Emily to think of conflict not as something to be afraid of, but as a chance to learn and grow. Sarah told Emily that picturing a successful outcome before having a hard conversation would help her feel more confident.

Sarah also suggested that Emily try deep breathing or other ways to relax to deal with her anxiety before talking to someone. To help Emily practice, they pretended to be in tense situations and Sarah gave Emily feedback on how she handled things.

Emily decided to talk about the problem with her team members because she felt better prepared. She set up a meeting and went over the conversation in her head, picturing it going well. She took a few deep breaths as she walked into the meeting room to calm her nerves.

During the meeting, Emily voiced her concerns in a clear and calm way. She focused on the facts and didn't make any personal attacks. She used techniques for "active listening," which gave her coworkers a chance to share their ideas and feelings. The team talked about what went wrong and came up with a plan to get the project back on track.

To Emily's surprise, the confrontation resulted in a more cohesive team, improved communication, and a successful project completion. Emily's professional relationships improved when she got over her fear of confrontation. She also grew as a person, realizing that being assertive was a valuable skill that helped her stand up for herself and others.

From then on, Emily kept practicing and getting better at being assertive, so she could face conflicts with confidence and understanding. She was able to handle difficult conversations with more grace after she learned how to do so. This helped her become a better project manager, creating a healthier workplace and better relationships with her team members.

· · · ● · ● · ● · ·

## Setting Healthy Boundaries

### Understanding the importance of personal boundaries

Personal boundaries are crucial for I/HSPs, as they allow us to protect our emotional and mental well-being. Personal boundaries can be thought of as the invisible lines we draw around ourselves to maintain a healthy sense of self and establish limits for how we interact with others. They serve as a critical aspect of self-care, helping to preserve our energy and ensure that our needs are met.

Below are some reasons why personal boundaries are essential for maintaining emotional and mental well-being:

1. **Establishing a sense of self-worth and self-respect:** Setting boundaries demonstrates that we value ourselves and our well-being. When we enforce our limits, we communicate to others that our needs and feelings are important, thereby fostering self-respect and self-worth.

2. **Preventing burnout and emotional exhaustion:** We are particularly susceptible to burnout and emotional exhaustion due to our tendency to absorb the emotions of others and require more downtime to recharge. Establishing boundaries helps protect our energy and allows us to prioritize self-care and recuperation.

3. **Fostering healthy relationships:** By setting and maintaining boundaries, we create a foundation for respectful, balanced relationships. Boundaries help ensure that our needs are met and that we're not overly accommodating the needs of others at our own expense. This mutual respect results in healthier, more fulfilling relationships.

4. **Managing stress and anxiety:** A lack of boundaries can lead to increased stress and anxiety, as we may find ourselves constantly trying to please others or worry about their reactions. Setting boundaries allows us to have greater control over our lives, reducing stress and anxiety levels.

5. **Promoting personal growth:** Establishing personal boundaries encourages introspection and self-awareness, as we must reflect on our needs, values, and limits to set effective boundaries. This process of self-discovery contributes to personal growth and development.

6. **Creating a safe space for self-expression:** When we have clear personal

boundaries, we create an environment where we can express ourselves openly and honestly without fear of judgment or criticism. This safe space allows us to explore our thoughts, feelings, and emotions, ultimately contributing to a healthier emotional and mental state.

Sophia, an HSP and introvert in her early 30s, had always struggled with setting personal boundaries. She often found herself saying yes to invitations, requests, and commitments that she didn't genuinely want to participate in, just to avoid disappointing others. She felt tired and overwhelmed by this constant need to make other people happy.

One day, after agreeing to attend yet another social event that she wasn't genuinely interested in, Sophia realized that her lack of personal boundaries was negatively affecting her mental and emotional well-being. She confided in her close friend, Laura, who had always been adept at maintaining healthy boundaries in her own life.

Laura told Sophia about her own experience and how important it was to have personal boundaries. She stressed that setting limits was not only good for Sophia's mental and emotional health, but was also important for building healthy relationships. She told Sophia to think about what she values, what she needs, and what her limits are, and to practice setting her limits in different situations.

Sophia took Laura's advice to heart and started putting herself first and setting her own limits. She started by turning down an invitation to a party because she needed time alone to rest. Sophia was worried about letting her friends down, but she was happy to find that they respected her decision and understood her need to take care of herself.

Sophia kept practicing setting limits after this, which gave her more confidence. She started saying no to work tasks that weren't part of her job description. This gave her the time and energy to focus on her main tasks without feeling too busy. She also told her family what she couldn't do and asked them to give her space and time alone when she needed it.

Over time, Sophia noticed that her mental and emotional health had gotten a lot better. She felt more in control of her life and experienced less stress and anxiety. Her relationships also got better because she was able to be more real with people and make connections where everyone respected each other.

Sophia's real-life situation shows how important it is to understand and set personal boundaries. By setting and maintaining healthy limits, she was able to protect her emotional and mental well-being, foster healthier relationships, and live a more balanced, fulfilling life.

· · · ● · ● · ● · ·

## Identifying and communicating your limits

1. **Reflect on your values and priorities:** Consider what is most important to you and identify any areas where you feel your boundaries have been crossed.

2. **Be specific and clear about your boundaries:** Clearly communicate your limits and expectations to others, both verbally and non-verbally.

3. **Be consistent:** Enforce your boundaries consistently, regardless of who is involved or the circumstances.

4. **Remember that it's okay to say "no":** Practice saying "no" without guilt or shame. Recognize that your needs and well-being are just as important as those of others.

Nathan, a 35-year-old introvert, had always had trouble saying "no" to other people, whether at work, with friends, or in his family life. He couldn't set limits because he was afraid of letting other people down and wanted to be seen as helpful and dependable. Unfortunately, his mental health and overall well-being were starting to suffer because he always said yes.

Nathan's coworkers quickly learned that he rarely said no to a request, so they often gave him tasks that were not part of his job. Because of this, he had a lot more work to do, so he worked late and felt stressed all the time.

In his personal life, Nathan agreed to go to a lot of social events, even though he was tired and needed time alone to rest. His friends and family liked how willing he was to help, but they didn't know how much pressure and stress he felt from always taking on too much.

Nathan's inability to say "no" started to show up in many different parts of his life. His work performance went downhill as he tried to keep up with an ever-growing list of tasks, and his manager gave him negative feedback about missed deadlines and a drop in productivity. Also, Nathan's relationships started to get tense because he was always tired and stressed, which made him cranky and less present in social situations.

After spending yet another late night at work, Nathan finally lost it. He realized that not being able to say "no" was making his life very hard and that he needed to change. He told Lily, a coworker who was known for being able to keep her work and personal life in balance. She understood Nathan's situation and told him about how hard it was for her to set limits in the past.

Lily told Nathan that he should start learning how to say "no" by making a list of his priorities and deciding if a request fits with those priorities. She told him to make his limits clear in a firm but polite way and to stop feeling bad about not being able to meet everyone's needs.

Taking Lily's advice, Nathan began to evaluate each request that came his way and consider whether he had the time, energy, and resources to commit to it. He slowly learned to say "no" to things that weren't his job or that got in the way of his self-care, work-life balance, and other personal goals.

Nathan's mental health, work performance, and relationships all got better over time after he learned how to set boundaries. By learning to say "no" when he needed to, he got back in charge of his life and was able to focus on the things that really mattered to him.

· · · ● ● · ● ● · ·

## Respecting the boundaries of others

1. **Ask for clarification:** If you're unsure about someone's boundaries, ask for clarification to avoid unintentional overstepping.

2. **Respect their wishes:** Honor the boundaries set by others, even if they differ from your own.

3. **Apologize and adjust when necessary:** If you unintentionally cross someone's boundaries, apologize and make a conscious effort to respect their limits moving forward.

· · · · ·•· ● · ●·•· · ·

# Managing Conflict and Difficult Situations

## Approaching conflicts with empathy and understanding

1. **Be mindful in your interactions:** Show genuine interest in the other person's perspective, and try to understand their feelings and needs.

2. **Validate their emotions:** Acknowledge and validate the other person's emotions without judgment or dismissal.

3. **Find common ground:** Identify shared goals or concerns to help bridge the gap between differing perspectives.

4. **Be open-minded and flexible:** Be willing to compromise and consider alternative solutions to resolve the conflict.

## Techniques for resolving disagreements

1. **Use the DESC model:** The DESC model stands for Describe, Express, Specify, and Consequences. This communication technique can be helpful in resolving disagreements by providing a structured approach to expressing your concerns and needs.

   ○ Describe the situation objectively and factually

   ○ Express your feelings and emotions about the situation

   ○ Specify what you would like to see changed or what you need

   ○ Explain the consequences, both positive and negative, of meeting or not meeting your request

In the following scenario, Amanda, a graphic designer, uses the DESC model to communicate with her coworker, Mark, about an issue with their collaborative project.

Amanda and Mark are working together on a marketing campaign for a major client. Amanda notices that Mark has consistently been submitting his work late, causing delays in the project timeline. She decides to address the issue using the DESC model.

**Describe**: *"Hey Mark, I noticed that over the past few weeks, the drafts for the marketing materials have been coming in later than our agreed-upon deadlines."*

**Express**: *"I feel concerned because the delays have been affecting my ability to complete my part of the project on time, and I'm worried we may miss our overall deadline."*

**Specify**: *"To ensure that we stay on track, could you please submit your drafts by the agreed-upon deadlines in the future? If there's any issue or if you need assistance, please let me know, and we can work together to find a solution."*

**Consequences**: *"By submitting your drafts on time, we can make sure that our project stays on schedule, and we can deliver a high-quality marketing campaign to our client."*

1. **Focus on the issue, not the person:** Address the specific problem or behavior, rather than making personal attacks or criticisms.

**Wrong way:**

In the following scenario, Emily, a project manager, addresses an issue with her team member, John, in an inappropriate manner.

Emily: *"John, you're always so disorganized and irresponsible. Your reports are consistently full of errors, and it's causing problems for the entire team. It's like you don't even care about the quality of your work."*

In this example, Emily focuses on John as a person, using personal attacks and criticisms instead of addressing the specific issue at hand. This approach is likely to make John feel defensive and resentful, leading to a breakdown in communication and a negative working relationship.

**Right way:**

Now, let's take a look at how Emily could have addressed the issue more effectively by focusing on the problem rather than the person.

Emily: *"John, I've noticed that some of the recent reports you've submitted have contained errors that needed to be corrected. It's essential for the team's efficiency and the quality of our work that we submit accurate reports. Can we discuss some strategies to help minimize these errors in the future?"*

In this revised example, Emily focuses on the specific issue—the errors in the reports—without making personal attacks or criticisms. By addressing the problem directly and offering to work together on a solution, Emily creates an atmosphere of collaboration and mutual respect, fostering a more positive and productive working relationship with John.

1. **Take breaks if needed:** If emotions are running high, it can be helpful to take a break and return to the conversation when both parties are calmer.

2. **Agree to disagree:** Recognize that it's not always possible to reach a resolution, and sometimes agreeing to disagree is the best course of action.

· · · ● · ● · · ·

# Handling criticism and feedback with grace

1. **Listen carefully:** Pay attention to the feedback and try to understand the other person's perspective, even if it's difficult to hear.

2. **Ask for clarification:** If you're unsure about the intent or specifics of the criticism, ask for more information to better understand the issue.

3. **Separate the message from the messenger:** Focus on the content of the feedback, rather than the person delivering it.

4. **Take time to process:** Give yourself time to process the criticism and consider how you can use it to grow and improve.

5. **Respond constructively:** Address the feedback by acknowledging any valid points and discussing how you plan to address them, while also standing up for yourself if you feel the criticism is unwarranted.

When you develop assertiveness skills, set healthy boundaries, and manage conflict with empathy and understanding, you can navigate the challenges of adulting with confidence and grace.

# CHAPTER TWELVE

## NURTURING YOUR SPIRITUAL LIFE

W E CAN SOMETIMES FEEL like we're swimming against the current in a world that is often loud, busy, and overwhelming. In the midst of chaos, it can be important to find a sense of inner peace and stability in order to handle life with grace and strength. Taking care of our spiritual lives can be a powerful way to find inner peace and learn more about who we are, what we value, and where we fit in the world.

This chapter will help you go on a journey to learn more about your spiritual life and grow as a person. We'll look into many different parts of spirituality, like personal beliefs and different spiritual practices, as well as how to use mindfulness and meditation in everyday life. Also, we'll talk about how connecting with nature and the environment can be healing, and how you can take care of the environment by doing things outside.

As you start this journey, keep in mind that there is no one right way to be spiritual. It is a very personal and unique experience, and your path will be different from everyone else's. It's important to go into this exploration with a sense of wonder, an open mind, and a desire to learn and grow. You might find that your spiritual journey improves not only your health but also your relationships, your creativity, and your life in a lot of other ways.

So, let's start this journey of self-discovery and spiritual growth and find out the many ways you can care for your spiritual life.

・ ・ ・ ● ・ ● ・ ● ・ ・ ・

## Exploring Spirituality and Personal Beliefs

### Reflecting on your values and beliefs

The process of introspection and the identification of guiding principles can be a source of comfort. To begin this journey, consider the following steps:

1. **Self-reflection:** Set aside some quiet time to reflect on your core beliefs and values. Journaling can be a helpful tool in this process. Write down your thoughts on topics such as your purpose in life, your understanding of a higher power or the universe, and your moral compass.

2. **Discussion with trusted individuals:** Engage in open and non-judgmental conversations with friends, family members, or mentors who share or have different beliefs. These discussions can help you gain new insights and refine your understanding of your own beliefs.

・ ・ ・ ● ・ ● ・ ● ・ ・ ・

## Investigating various spiritual practices and traditions

Broadening your understanding of different spiritual practices and traditions can enrich your spiritual journey. Consider researching the following:

- World religions, such as Christianity, Islam, Hinduism, Buddhism, and Judaism

- Eastern philosophies, such as Taoism and Confucianism

- Indigenous spiritual practices

- New Age spirituality and Mysticism

- Secular humanism and atheism

It's important to maintain an open mind, curiosity, and a healthy dose of respect as you learn about and engage with new cultural practices. Keep in mind that your beliefs and practices can evolve over time.

. . . . ● . ● . . .

# Developing a personal philosophy

As you learn more about different spiritual practices and beliefs, you will start to form your own personal philosophy. This way of thinking can help you grow spiritually and guide your actions and decisions. When forming your own philosophy, think about the following:

- What beliefs and values resonate with you the most?

- Are there any practices or rituals that you find meaningful and helpful?

- How does your personal philosophy align with your identity as an introvert or HSP?

Remember that developing a personal philosophy is an ongoing process, and it's okay to change and improve your beliefs as you continue to grow and learn.

. . . . ● . ● . . .

# Mindfulness and Meditation

### The benefits of mindfulness for I/HSPs

Mindfulness exercises are useful because they boost our psychological and emotional health. Some benefits of mindfulness include:

- Reduced stress and anxiety

- Enhanced self-awareness

- Improved emotional regulation

- Greater resilience in the face of challenges

- Deepened connections with others

• • • ●• ●• • •

## Different types of meditation practices

As mentioned in Chapter 6, there are various meditation practices that you can incorporate into your daily routine. Some popular types include:

**1. Breath-focused meditation**

Breath-focused meditation involves concentrating on the sensation of your breath as it moves in and out of your body. This practice encourages you to anchor your attention on the natural rhythm of your breath, which can help calm your mind and reduce stress. To practice breath-focused meditation:

- Find a comfortable seated position.

- Close your eyes and take a few deep breaths.

- Allow your breath to return to its natural rhythm.

- Focus your attention on the sensation of the air entering and leaving your nostrils or the rise and fall of your chest.

- If your mind wanders, gently bring your attention back to your breath.

**2. Body scan meditation**

Body scan meditation involves progressively scanning your body for sensations, tension, and relaxation. This practice can help you develop greater body awareness and release physical tension. To practice body scan meditation:

- Lie down comfortably on your back with your arms at your sides.

- Close your eyes and take a few deep breaths.

- Begin at your feet and gradually move your attention up through your body, noticing any sensations, tension, or relaxation in each area.

- As you focus on each body part, consciously release any tension you find.

- Continue scanning until you reach the top of your head.

## 3. Loving-kindness meditation

Loving-kindness meditation, also known as "metta" meditation, involves cultivating feelings of love and compassion towards yourself and others. This practice can help improve your relationships, boost self-compassion, and increase positive emotions. To practice loving-kindness meditation:

- Find a comfortable seated position.

- Close your eyes and take a few deep breaths.

- Silently repeat phrases such as "May I be happy, may I be healthy, may I be safe, may I be at ease."

- After a few minutes, shift your focus to someone you love and repeat the phrases for them.

- Gradually expand your focus to include friends, acquaintances, and even people with whom you have difficulties.

- Finally, extend your loving kindness to all beings everywhere.

## 4. Visualization meditation

Visualization meditation involves using mental imagery to promote relaxation or manifest positive outcomes. This practice can help reduce stress, enhance creativity, and increase feelings of empowerment. To practice visualization meditation:

- Find a comfortable seated or lying position.

- Close your eyes and take a few deep breaths.

- Imagine a peaceful scene or situation, such as a beautiful beach, a lush forest, or a moment of personal triumph.

- Engage all your senses in this imagined scene, noting the sights, sounds, smells, tastes, and physical sensations.

- Allow yourself to fully experience the positive emotions associated with the visualization.

## 5. Mantra meditation

Mantra meditation involves repeating a word or phrase, such as "Om" or "peace," to maintain focus and calm the mind. This practice can help quiet mental chatter, increase concentration, and induce relaxation. To practice mantra meditation:

- Find a comfortable seated position.

- Close your eyes and take a few deep breaths.

- Choose a word or phrase that has personal meaning or significance to you.

- Silently repeat your chosen mantra, either in coordination with your breath or at a steady rhythm.

- If your mind wanders, gently bring your attention back to the repetition of your mantra.

Experiment with different techniques to find the one that works best for you.

• • • • ● • ● • • •

# Incorporating mindfulness into daily life

Mindfulness is the practice of becoming aware of your thoughts, feelings, and body sensations in each moment, as well as your surroundings. By making mindfulness a part of your everyday life, you can get a lot of benefits, such as less stress and anxiety, better focus, and better emotional health. Here are some easy ways to bring mindfulness into your daily life, along with tips from Thich Nhat Hanh, a Buddhist monk and mindfulness teacher from Vietnam:

### 1. Set aside a specific time each day for meditation or mindfulness practice

Getting into the habit of being mindful can be helped by doing the same thing every day. Choose a time that works best for you, whether it's in the morning, during your lunch break, or before you go to sleep. As much as possible, try to stick to this schedule to help you get into the habit.

### 2. Use apps or guided meditation recordings to support your practice

There are many mindfulness apps and guided meditation recordings that can help you with your practice and help you get more out of it. These resources can help you develop mindfulness by giving you advice, ideas, and structure. Some popular mindfulness apps include Headspace, Calm, and Insight Timer.

### 3. Incorporate mindfulness into everyday activities

Thich Nhat Hanh talks a lot about how important it is to be fully present when doing everyday things, turning them into mindful experiences. Here are some ways to practice being mindful every day:

- **Mindful walking:** Focus on the sensations of your feet touching the ground, the rhythm of your breath, and the movement of your body as you walk.

- **Mindful eating:** Savor each bite of food, paying attention to its taste, texture, and aroma. Eat slowly and appreciate the nourishment it provides.

- **Mindful cleaning:** As you wash dishes, sweep the floor, or clean your living space, focus on the physical sensations and the act of making your environment more pleasant.

### 4. Attend local meditation or mindfulness workshops and classes

Connecting with people who share your interest in mindfulness can give you support, encouragement, and a sense of community. Find meditation or mindfulness workshops, classes, or retreats in your area where you can learn new skills, share your own experiences, and build a community of people who practice mindfulness.

### 5. Embrace Thich Nhat Hanh's teachings on mindful breathing

Thich Nhat Hanh teaches that breathing with awareness is a powerful way to develop awareness and peace of mind. He says that paying attention to your breath can help you stay in the present and give you a break from the chaos of everyday life. To breathe mindfully, all you have to do is:

- Inhale deeply, being aware of the sensation of the breath entering your body.

- Exhale fully, releasing any tension or stress as you breathe out.

- Continue to focus on your breath, allowing thoughts and distractions to come and go without judgment.

· · · ● ● · ● · · ·

## Connecting with Nature and the Environment

### The healing power of nature

For those of us who need a break from the constant stimulation of modern life and a chance to refuel, nature can be a haven. The healing power of nature includes:

- Reduced stress and anxiety

- Improved mood and emotional well-being

- Increased creativity and problem-solving abilities

- Greater connection to the natural world and its rhythms

**Engaging in outdoor activities and hobbies**

Think about doing hobbies and outdoor activities that match your interests and energy levels. Some possibilities include:

- Hiking and nature walks

- Gardening and plant care

- Birdwatching and wildlife observation

- Outdoor photography or painting

- Picnics and outdoor reading

Remember to respect your personal boundaries and energy levels, and choose activities that genuinely resonate with you.

**Practicing environmental stewardship and sustainability**

As you get closer to nature, think about ways to be a good environmental steward and support sustainability. Some ideas include:

- Reducing waste and recycling

- Conserving water and energy at home

- Supporting local and organic food sources

- Participating in community clean-ups or conservation projects

- Advocating for environmental protection and sustainable practices

You can live a balanced and fulfilling life by taking care of your spiritual life, practicing mindfulness, and spending time in nature. Remember that your spiritual journey is personal and ever-evolving, and it's essential to approach it with curiosity, openness, and self-compassion.

# CHAPTER THIRTEEN

## BUILDING CONFIDENCE AND OVERCOMING SELF-DOUBT

A DULTING IS DIFFICULT FOR everyone, but for us, it can feel especially overwhelming. The world around us often seems like it was made for people who like to be around other people and be "on" all the time. It's understandable that feelings of insecurity and uncertainty would arise in such a setting. But don't worry! This section is meant to help you feel better about yourself, so you can embrace your individuality and excel in all areas of your life.

Confidence is not a destination; it's a journey. It's an ongoing process of getting to know yourself, being kind to yourself, and growing as a person. Whether you're just starting your adulting journey or you're looking to further develop your self-confidence, this chapter will provide you with the tools and insights you need to cultivate a healthy self-image and navigate the world with confidence.

In this chapter, we'll get into the details of how to recognize your inner critic and how to stop yourself from saying bad things to yourself. I'll talk about how important it is to have a growth mindset and be proud of what makes you unique. I'll also give you ways to set goals that you can reach, be kind to yourself, and embrace your true self.

Through real-life stories and advice from experts, we'll look at the successes and failures I/HSPs have had on their way to becoming more confident. These stories remind you that you're not alone on your journey, and they also give you ideas and tips for getting over self-doubt.

So, let's embark on a life-changing adventure that will ultimately lead to higher levels of self-assurance. The information in this chapter will help you recognize your own value and stop doubting your abilities. Let's get going!

• • • ● • ● • • •

## Recognizing Your Inner Critic

### Identifying self-defeating thoughts and beliefs

Being aware of our own personal inner critic is crucial for people like us. This inner voice often tells us thoughts and beliefs that make us feel bad about ourselves and keep us from reaching our full potential. Some common examples of self-defeating thoughts are:

- "I'm not good enough."

- "I can't do it."

- "Nobody likes me."

To overcome these thoughts, try the following techniques:

1. **Keep a thought journal:** Write down any negative thoughts that come up throughout the day. By becoming aware of these thoughts, you'll be better equipped to challenge them.

2. **Identify patterns:** Look for common themes in your negative thoughts. Are they related to specific situations or people? Recognizing patterns can help you address the root causes of your self-doubt.

Sarah, a 28-year-old graphic designer and classic introvert, has always been more comfortable working alone and spending her free time reading or doing her favorite things. Sarah has been having trouble with self-doubt, especially in social situations and networking events. She has noticed that she often feels anxious and overwhelmed in these situations and has been having negative thoughts like "I'm not interesting enough" or "I'm too awkward."

Sarah wanted to face her self-doubt head-on, so she decided to keep a thought journal for a month. Every time she had a bad thought, she would write it down along with the situation or people she was thinking about. As Sarah read through her journal entries, she started to notice a pattern: most of her bad thoughts came up at social events or when she was with her outgoing coworkers.

When Sarah noticed this pattern, she decided to dig deeper to find out what was making her doubt herself. She came to understand that her anxiety was a result of her concern about other people's opinions of her and the pressure to blend in with an outgoing society. Armed with this knowledge, Sarah took steps to change her way of thinking and come up with ways to deal with situations like these.

Sarah first started doing mindfulness exercises to help her stay in the moment and grounded at social events. She also started going to smaller gatherings and meetups that were geared toward her interests. There, she met people who were just like her and who liked how shy she was. Sarah also joined an online support group for introverts. This gave her a safe place to talk about her problems and learn from others who were going through the same things.

Over time, Sarah noticed that her negative thoughts got a lot better and that her self-confidence went up. Sarah was able to overcome her self-doubt and be proud of her unique qualities as an introvert by figuring out the patterns in her negative thoughts and dealing with the reasons behind them.

· · · ● · ● · · ·

## Challenging negative self-talk

Once you've identified your self-defeating thoughts, it's time to challenge them. Here are some ways to do that:

- **Ask for evidence:** When a negative thought pops up, ask yourself, "What's the evidence for this thought?" More often than not, you'll find that there's little to no evidence to support your inner critic's claims.

- **Reframe your thoughts:** Instead of accepting your negative thoughts at face value, try to reframe them in a more positive light. For example, if you think, "I can't do this," reframe it as, "This is a challenge, but I can learn and grow from it."

· · · ● · ● · ● · · ·

## Cultivating a growth mindset

Developing a growth mindset is key to overcoming self-doubt. A growth mindset is the belief that your abilities can be developed through dedication and hard work. To cultivate a growth mindset:

- **Embrace challenges:** See challenges as opportunities for growth, rather than obstacles.

- **Celebrate effort, not just results:** Recognize the value of hard work and perseverance, even if the outcome isn't perfect.

- **Learn from setbacks:** Instead of viewing setbacks as failures, see them as valuable learning experiences.

· · · ● · ● · ● · · ·

## Embracing Your Unique Qualities

### Celebrating your strengths and talents

Your skills and abilities are one of a kind. Some of these might be the ability to think deeply, be creative, have empathy, and make connections that matter. Recognize these traits by:

- **Making a list:** Write down all of your strengths and talents, and keep it somewhere you can see it often.

- **Sharing your gifts:** Use your strengths and talents to help others or contribute to a cause you're passionate about.

· • • ● • ● • • ·

## Acknowledging your accomplishments

Recognize and celebrate your accomplishments, big and small. This can help build your confidence and remind you of your capabilities. To do this:

- **Keep a "brag file":** Keep a record of your achievements, compliments, and positive feedback from others.

- **Celebrate your wins:** Take time to acknowledge and celebrate your successes, whether it's a completed project, a personal milestone, or even just a small victory.

· • ● • ● • • ·

## Overcoming the fear of judgment and rejection

It's normal to be afraid of being misunderstood or rejected. To overcome this fear:

- **Practice self-compassion:** Be kind to yourself and remember that everyone experiences fear and self-doubt at times.

- **Focus on your values:** Align your actions with your core values, and remind yourself that the opinions of others don't define your worth.

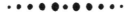

## Developing Confidence and Self-Trust

Setting achievable goals and working toward them

Building confidence requires setting realistic, achievable goals and working toward them. By doing this, you'll develop a sense of accomplishment and self-efficacy. To set achievable goals:

1. **Break goals into smaller steps:** Breaking a big goal into smaller, more manageable steps makes it easier to tackle and helps you see progress along the way.

2. **Set SMART goals:** Make sure your goals are Specific, Measurable, Achievable, Relevant, and Time-bound.

3. **Celebrate progress:** Acknowledge and celebrate the progress you make toward your goals, even if it's incremental.

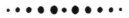

## Practicing self-compassion and self-forgiveness

Self-compassion is the act of showing yourself the same compassion you would give to a close friend. To practice self-compassion:

- **Mindfulness:** Be aware of your thoughts and feelings without judgment, and accept them as they are.

- **Common humanity:** Recognize that everyone makes mistakes and faces challenges. You are not alone in your struggles.

- **Self-kindness:** Offer yourself kindness and understanding when faced with setbacks or mistakes.

Just as it's important to forgive others, it's equally important to forgive ourselves. Forgiving oneself entails releasing the guilt and resentment that come from realizing past errors. To practice self-forgiveness:

- **Acknowledge your mistakes:** Accept that you've made mistakes, but don't let them define you.

- **Learn from your mistakes:** Reflect on what you can learn from past errors and how you can apply these lessons moving forward.

- **Let go of guilt and shame:** Release negative feelings associated with your mistakes and focus on your growth and progress.

· · · ● · ● · · ·

## Embracing your authentic self

Recognize and value what makes you who you are if you want to feel secure in your own skin. Here are some ways to do this:

- **Know your values:** Understand what's important to you and make decisions based on your core values.

- **Be true to yourself:** Don't try to fit into someone else's mold or conform to societal expectations. Instead, embrace your individuality and authenticity.

- **Find your tribe:** Surround yourself with people who appreciate and support your authentic self.

If you put these methods into practice, you'll soon find that you have more confidence and less self-doubt. Keep in mind that developing your sense of self-worth takes time and effort. Don't give up on yourself and keep going.

# CHAPTER FOURTEEN

# TIME MANAGEMENT AND ORGANIZATION FOR I/HSPS

B EING AN INTROVERT MYSELF, I can relate to the stress of trying to stay on top of everything and still get everything done. I mean, let's be honest: adulting can be hard. In fact, I've been known to procrastinate so much that my to-do list has its own to-do list! And don't get me started on multi-tasking. I once attempted to cook dinner, answer work emails, and watch a documentary on sloths simultaneously. Spoiler alert: it wasn't pretty. Burnt pasta, typos, and an incomplete understanding of sloth ecology were the results of my multitasking adventure.

And then there's my desk. It's like a scene from one of those "Where's Waldo?" books, except instead of Waldo, you're trying to find my stapler amidst a sea of papers, coffee mugs, and an impressive collection of pens that have long since run out of ink. It's a masterpiece of chaos that could give any modern art installation a run for its money.

As I've journeyed through this crazy thing called adulting, I've come to realize that time management and organization are crucial for I/HSPs like us. Not only do they help us stay on top of our tasks, but they also provide a sense of calm and stability in a world that often feels overwhelming. So, join me as we dive into the world of prioritizing, decluttering, and embracing effective routines in this chapter. Together, we'll tackle the art of adulting one task at a time, creating a more balanced, organized, and fulfilling life. And who knows, maybe by the end of this chapter, we'll finally be able to locate that elusive stapler!

• • • ● • ● • ● • •

## Prioritizing Tasks and Goals

Creating a realistic to-do list

- **Be honest with yourself:** Consider how much time you truly have available and what tasks you can realistically complete within that time frame.

- **Break it down:** Divide larger tasks into smaller, more manageable parts.

- **Prioritize:** Rank your tasks by importance or deadline, tackling the most critical items first.

John, an introverted accountant, sat with a stack of papers around him on another boring Monday morning. Determined to take charge of his day, he reached for his notebook and began crafting a to-do list. With a focus on maximizing productivity and accomplishing his tasks efficiently, John carefully prioritized his responsibilities.

John crossed off each item on the list as he worked his way through it. This gave him a sense of accomplishment. By setting priorities, he was able to approach his work with clarity and purpose, which made him more productive all day.

By the end of the workday, John was amazed that he had been able to do everything on his list. He was happy to think about how organizing and prioritizing his work had helped him.

From that day on, John continued to use to-do lists because he knew they could help him organize and get things done in his daily life. This new habit gave him a renewed sense of control and the ability to get things done on Mondays and during the workweek.

• • • ● • ● • ● • •

## Establishing short-term and long-term goals

- **Short-term goals:** Identify achievable objectives that you can accomplish within a few weeks or months.

- **Long-term goals:** Consider your long-term aspirations, such as career growth or personal development, and set goals with a timeline of several years.

Jessica, a talented and highly sensitive freelance writer, carried a deep-seated dream within her—to publish her own novel. She was passionate and determined, and she knew that to reach her goal, she had to stay focused and motivated.

To navigate the demanding journey of writing a book, Jessica implemented a strategic approach. She set both short-term and long-term goals to guide her progress. In the short term, she aimed to write a certain number of words per week, steadily chipping away at her manuscript. Simultaneously, she set her sights on the long-term objective of completing her entire manuscript within two years.

Finally, after years of diligent work, Jessica's efforts paid off. She achieved her ultimate dream and proudly published her novel, "The Introvert's Guide to Surviving a Zombie Apocalypse." (Note: This is not a real book, but we can imagine the premise!)

· · · · ● · ● · · ·

## Breaking down tasks into manageable steps

- Identify the main components of a task.

- Assign a time frame for each step.

- Monitor your progress and adjust your plan as needed.

When Carlos, an introverted software engineer, was handed a daunting project, his initial reaction was a mixture of excitement and dread. As he gazed at the complexity of the task, a wave of overwhelm threatened to consume him. But Carlos wasn't one to back down from a challenge.

Taking a deep breath and channeling his inner Zen master, Carlos devised a plan to conquer the project without succumbing to panic. He donned his coding cape and broke down the mammoth undertaking into bite-sized chunks. Writing specific sections of code became like solving a puzzle, one line at a time.

As the days turned into weeks, Carlos's focus and dedication paid off. He conquered each task with the precision of a ninja coder, meticulously running tests and ironing out bugs along the way. The project gradually took shape, like a digital masterpiece emerging from the depths of his imagination.

As he presented his completed work to his boss, Carlos's nerves transformed into a quiet confidence. His introverted nature hadn't hindered him—it had fueled his focus and attention to detail. His boss's eyes widened with awe and appreciation, recognizing Carlos's triumph over the monumental task.

· · · ●·●·●·● · ·

## Balancing Work and Personal Life

Allocating time for self-care and relaxation

- Schedule regular breaks throughout the day to recharge.

- Incorporate activities that bring you joy and relaxation, such as reading, meditation, or spending time in nature.

Jenny, a dedicated and empathetic teacher, found herself teetering on the edge of exhaustion and burnout from the demands of her job. Determined to regain her balance and well-being, she made a conscious decision to introduce short but meaningful breaks into her workday.

During these precious moments, Jenny prioritized self-care and nourishment for her soul. She practiced mindfulness, immersing herself in the present moment and allowing her mind to find serenity amidst the chaos. She listened to calming music that washed away the stress and rejuvenated her spirit. And she ventured outside, taking leisurely walks in the park, allowing nature's embrace to invigorate her senses.

As Jenny committed to these simple yet powerful changes, she witnessed a remarkable transformation within herself. She started to feel more energized and zestful for life as the exhaustion that had been weighing her down started to fade. With a restored spirit, she became not only a more effective educator but also a beacon of inspiration for her students.

Jenny's journey serves as a reminder to all that in the pursuit of nurturing others, we must never forget to nourish ourselves. By making intentional self-care a priority, we not only unlock our own potential but also become catalysts for positive change in the lives of those we touch.

· • • •●•●•• ·

## Managing distractions and interruptions

- Identify your personal distractions and develop strategies to minimize them.

- Communicate your needs and boundaries to others, politely requesting that they respect your focused time.

Tim, a talented and introverted graphic designer, found himself grappling with an all-too-familiar challenge—an open-concept office filled with constant distractions. Determined to reclaim his focus and productivity, he took matters into his own hands.

Armed with a pair of noise-canceling headphones, Tim entered his creative sanctuary. To reinforce the importance of uninterrupted concentration, he crafted a sign that read, "In the zone: please do not disturb." With a touch of humor and clear communication, Tim sent a powerful message to his colleagues about his need for quiet focus.

As his coworkers began to understand and respect his boundaries, a remarkable transformation occurred. The distractions that once hindered Tim's workflow faded into the background. Freed from interruptions, his creativity flourished, and his productivity skyrocketed.

Tim's decision to advocate for his needs demonstrated the power of setting boundaries and communicating them effectively. By taking proactive measures, he created an environment that nurtured his introverted nature, allowing his talents to shine.

• • • ● • ● • • •

## Establishing boundaries between work and home

- Set clear guidelines for when you are "on" and "off" work.

- Create physical and mental separation between your work and personal life, such as designating a specific workspace or having a post-work relaxation ritual.

Amelia, a highly sensitive remote employee, initially struggled to separate her work and personal life. To establish boundaries, she created a dedicated home office and established a strict schedule for work hours. After clocking out, Amelia would take a short walk to "commute" back to her personal life, signaling the end of her workday. This routine helped Amelia maintain a healthy work-life balance and avoid burnout.

• • ● • ● • • •

## Developing Effective Organization Skills

Tips for organizing your physical space

- **Declutter regularly:** Keep your workspace tidy by regularly discarding or organizing unnecessary items.

- **Organize by importance:** Arrange items based on how frequently you use them, keeping essentials within easy reach.

Chloe, an introverted librarian, was known for her messy desk. Determined to create a more organized workspace, she purged old documents, invested in some stylish organizers, and arranged her desk according to her daily needs. The result? A workspace that even Marie Kondo would approve of.

• • • • • • • • • •

## Utilizing digital tools and apps for organization

- **Explore productivity apps:** Experiment with digital tools such as task managers, note-taking apps, and calendar applications to find the best fit for your needs.

- **Sync your devices:** Ensure your organization system is accessible across all your devices to maintain consistency and convenience.

Pedro, a highly sensitive project manager, was juggling multiple deadlines and struggling to stay organized. After researching various digital tools, he discovered a task management app that changed his life. Pedro could now track his assignments, deadlines, and progress all in one place, syncing everything to his devices. Suddenly, adulting wasn't so hard anymore.

• • • • • • • • • •

## Creating routines and habits for productivity

- **Establish a daily routine:** Create a predictable daily schedule that includes time for work, self-care, and relaxation.

- **Develop productive habits:** Identify habits that boost your productivity and incorporate them into your daily routine.

Cassie, an introverted software developer, had trouble staying productive throughout her day. She decided to create a daily routine that started with a morning workout, followed by a healthy breakfast, and focused work sessions with scheduled breaks. By incorporating these productive habits into her daily routine, Cassie became more efficient and energized, ultimately enjoying her work and personal life more.

• • • • • • • • • •

## Different Time Management Techniques: Finding the One that Tickles Your Fancy

Throughout the years, I've tried various time management techniques in search of the Holy Grail of productivity. Some of them worked, some of them didn't, and some of them left me wondering if I had accidentally enrolled in a cult. But, like Goldilocks, I kept searching for the one that felt just right. And along the way, I discovered some pretty interesting methods that might tickle your fancy. Let's dive in!

### The Pomodoro Technique: For Those Who Love Tomatoes and Timers

The Pomodoro Technique is named after the tomato-shaped kitchen timer that its creator used. It involves breaking up your work into 25-minute chunks (called Pomodoros) with 5-minute breaks in between. After you've done four Pomodoros, you can give yourself a 15- to 30-minute break. It's perfect for people who like to race against the clock and like getting things done in ways that are inspired by Italian food.

### The Eisenhower Matrix: When You Need a General's Touch

The Eisenhower Matrix, which was named after President Dwight D. Eisenhower, helps you put tasks in order based on how important and how quickly they need to be done. The matrix has four quadrants: urgent and important, important but not urgent, urgent but not important, and neither urgent nor important. By categorizing your tasks this way, you can focus on what truly matters and avoid getting bogged down in the swamp of unimportant tasks that just love to eat up your time.

### The Two-Minute Rule: Because Who Doesn't Love Instant Gratification?

If a task can be completed in two minutes or less, just do it! This straightforward rule, made popular by David Allen's "Getting Things Done" (GTD) method, aids in clearing out those bothersome little tasks that frequently pile up and haunt your to-do list like tiny, annoying poltergeists. Suddenly, you're a time management superhero, eliminating tasks left and right with lightning speed!

## Getting Things Done (GTD): My Personal Favorite for Tackling Time Management

Now, let's talk about my all-time favorite technique, "Getting Things Done" by David Allen. GTD is like the Swiss Army knife of time management systems—it's got a tool for everything! The GTD method involves five key steps: capture, clarify, organize, reflect, and engage.

1. **Capture:** Jot down everything that's occupying your mind – tasks, ideas, reminders – and get them into a trusted system.

2. **Clarify:** Process each item, deciding if it's actionable, and if so, what the next action should be.

3. **Organize:** Sort your tasks into appropriate categories, such as projects, delegated tasks, or items to tackle at a later date.

4. **Reflect:** Regularly review your system, ensuring it's up to date and relevant.

5. **Engage:** With your tasks organized and prioritized, confidently choose your next action and get to work!

GTD has become my go-to method for time management because it feels like a loving, organized hug from the productivity gods. Plus, it's so comprehensive that I'm pretty sure David Allen has thought of everything, including how to handle that half-eaten sandwich that's been lurking at the back of your fridge for a suspiciously long time.

So, there you have it—an overview of some popular time management techniques that could bring a much-needed chuckle and perhaps even revolutionize your productivity game. Whether you're a fan of tomatoes, matrixes, instant gratification, or embracing your inner productivity ninja, there's a method out there that will suit your unique sensibilities. Happy time managing!

# Epilogue

AND SO, WE HAVE reached the end of our journey through the thrilling, sometimes chaotic, but always rewarding world of adulting. We've debunked myths, navigated relationships, conquered our finances, prioritized self-care, and even managed to find our staplers. Together, we've laughed, we've cried, and we've learned that adulting, while challenging, is a journey worth taking.

As we say goodbye to this book and to each other, I want to leave you with a few golden nuggets of wisdom that you can take with you as you continue adulting.

1. **Embrace your introverted and highly sensitive nature.** Remember, you possess unique strengths and qualities that make you who you are. You're not just a wallflower; you're a rare and exotic orchid, thriving in your own way.

2. **Adulting is an ongoing process.** It's okay if you don't have everything figured out right now. Even the most "adult" adults are still learning and growing. So give yourself a break, and remember that Rome wasn't built in a day – and neither were you.

3. **Don't be afraid to ask for help.** We are not alone. Reach out to friends, family, or even a professional when you need support. Trust me, they won't bite (unless they're going through a weird zombie phase).

4. **Celebrate your successes, no matter how small.** Did you finally manage to fold a fitted sheet without it turning into a lumpy, misshapen blob?

Congratulations! You've just unlocked the "Domestic Wizard" achievement. Be proud of your accomplishments and let them fuel your motivation for future adulting endeavors.

5. **Remember that life is meant to be enjoyed.** While adulting can be stressful and overwhelming at times, don't forget to make room for laughter, joy, and the occasional dance party in your living room. After all, life's too short not to bust a move every once in a while.

As we part ways, I hope you take these lessons to heart and continue to adult hard, one step at a time. May your journey be full of learning, strength, and a good dose of humor. And always remember that you're not alone when you feel lost or overwhelmed. We're all just trying to figure it out, one awkward social interaction and misfiled tax return at a time.

Now, go forth and conquer! The world may not always understand us, but together, we'll show them that we're more than capable of navigating this wild ride called adulting, and we'll do it with grace, finesse, and a heaping spoonful of laughter.

Here's to you, the I/HSPs of the world, for being the unsung heroes of adulting. May your days be filled with quiet moments, deep connections, and an abundance of perfectly organized desk drawers.

Thank you!

Jeff

# PLEASE CONSIDER LEAVING A REVIEW

Hello there!

As an author, I know just how important reviews are for getting the word out about my work. When readers leave a review on Amazon, it helps others discover my book and decide whether it's right for them.

Plus, it gives me valuable feedback on what readers enjoyed and what they didn't.

So if you've read my book and enjoyed it (or even if you didn't!), I would really appreciate it if you took a moment to leave a review on Amazon. It doesn't have to be long or complicated - just a few words about what you thought of the book would be incredibly helpful.

Thank you so much for your support!


Jeff

# ALSO BY

**Adulting Hard for Young Men**

**Adulting Hard for Young Women**